KICK
DEPRESSION
IN THE
GUTS

ROSS WILKINSON (B.E.)

Dr Monica Wilkinson (PhD.)

The**Book**Studio

All correspondence to the author:

Email: rosswilko@bigpond.com
Facebook: blackdogtoolbox

ISBN: 978-0-646-8221-5-0

Proudly produced by

TheBookStudio
www.thebookstudio.com.au

CONTENTS

Introduction

When I started writing this book in April 2019, I wasn't going to have an Introduction. I really wanted page 1 to be my solutions to Depression. Open up the book and then BANG, the answers would be there.

If you want to read the Intro then go and do what I suggest, without buying my book, what do I care? It's also because I rarely read introductions myself, but I'm informed that others do. I have written this for you, the people that do read Introductions.

When I was a boy at a Christian school, I could never get my head around the Jesus thing. Why talk to the 2IC (Jesus) when you can go straight to the boss? You know what I mean; I just want answers, I don't want to go through an intermediary.

If I go to McDonalds (which I don't) it's because I'm hungry and I want a burger. (You would have to be hungry to eat that stuff). The fries, shakes, and toys are all fluff as far as I'm concerned. I am not going to try to market to you. You are clever enough to decide for yourself whether I am sincere, and whether you should waste your time and money on this book. I am not here to grab your attention, or to make big bucks (though it would be nice). I'm here to tell you what worked for me and why it will work for you. So here are my reasons for, and solutions to your Depression. I am not a professional author, which will become obvious as we progress, if you haven't realised already.

1. Antibiotics are the number one cause of Depression. The great thing about this theory is that you are not to blame. There is no guilt to this. You took something that was good for your health and it had side effects. Unfortunately, now you have to solve it, you have to solve your gut health. Why are antibiotics the culprit? It's because antibiotics not only kill bad bacteria, but good bacteria too. You probably didn't know you had good bacteria but you do;

you have trillions of them - literally. When you kill lots of them off accidentally or intentionally, trouble begins.

2. Diet...no free ride here, except that many of the things you have been told about diet, have little evidence to support them, or are just plain wrong. That doesn't mean you need to eat mung beans or go vegetarian. Just lay off the junk food please, even if it's just until you solve your Depression.

3. Loss of nature (the outdoors) and natural foods in your diet. Again, you don't have to go organic, vegetarian, or swan around at the nude beach, but a bit of digging in the garden, sunshine, traditional meat and three-veg meal (plus a bit of sauerkraut) will do just fine.

Sounds too simple? Maybe, but it's a lot easier and cheaper than sitting on a couch for hours getting in touch with your inner self. Or paying some guru or highly trained professional. It's a lot easier than meditating, or yoga, or finding the meaning of life. Maybe I'm wrong (I'm not, because I did it myself) but what I suggest could be worth a try.

There is certainly no shame in not having previous knowledge of the things I am about to tell you. The science behind what you're about to learn is fairly new. The concepts are ancient, but the science is new.

I sincerely hope to blow your mind, and not bore you.

If that helps sell this book, good for me. If it doesn't, I will live with that.

I won't tell you to do anything and I will not wag my finger at you. I just want you to get out of this shitful situation. I've been there, and now I'm free. It didn't take me long and I didn't have to become a monk or find the meaning of life. Oh, and I didn't write this book for the millions of people that want to help you or cure you. I wrote it for you, the person with Depression. Plenty of people will tell me that I'm full of it, or don't know what I'm doing...fair enough, but who cares what they think?

This book is not for them, it's for <u>YOU</u> (and anyone you love or care about who's battling with Depression).

This isn't a 'touchy feely' book, nor was it designed for the politically correct among you. If you don't like a bit of profanity, a few jokes, or being challenged about the accepted norms surrounding Depression, you've been warned that the contents may not be your cup of tea.

If you prefer to dot your 'i's and cross your 't's, again, maybe it's not for you. As Doc says to Marty in *Back to the Future 1*... *"Please excuse the crudity of this model, it's not to scale and I didn't have time to paint it."*

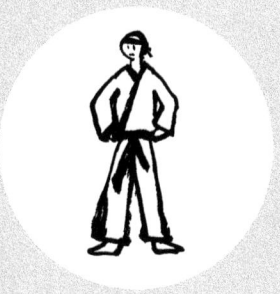

PART 1

HOW TO FIX DEPRESSION
+ ABOUT ME

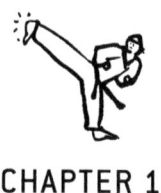

CHAPTER 1

Fixing Your Depression

Why is this book called **Kick Depression in the Guts**? Because it's about solving your Depression problems using simple techniques and in particular, fixing your gut health. There are heaps of scientific studies that support this theory. I didn't consult these studies to cure my Depression. I fixed it first and then I found the studies later. I won't waste your time, and I won't get you to do weird stuff, just simple, everyday, practical solutions - Good luck!

I'm an engineer. Engineers fix stuff (mostly). They fix problems then delve into the 'why' later. I think that's my new motto: Shoot first, ask questions later.

I am here to fix your Depression, just like I fixed mine. I will tell you how in this chapter and you can find out why later, if you're interested. If you're not, that's fine with me. Not everyone wants explanations. Some people just want answers, and that's okay.

It will cost you hardly any money. I mean you bought this book, so you might as well read it. Maybe I have your solution, maybe not, but I'm pretty sure I do. I don't deal in certainty though. I'm sort of an 80 to 90% guy. That will do me. After you fix your Depression you may have other psychological issues to solve, like stress management, or assertiveness, or finding the meaning of life. I can't fix those psychological issues that

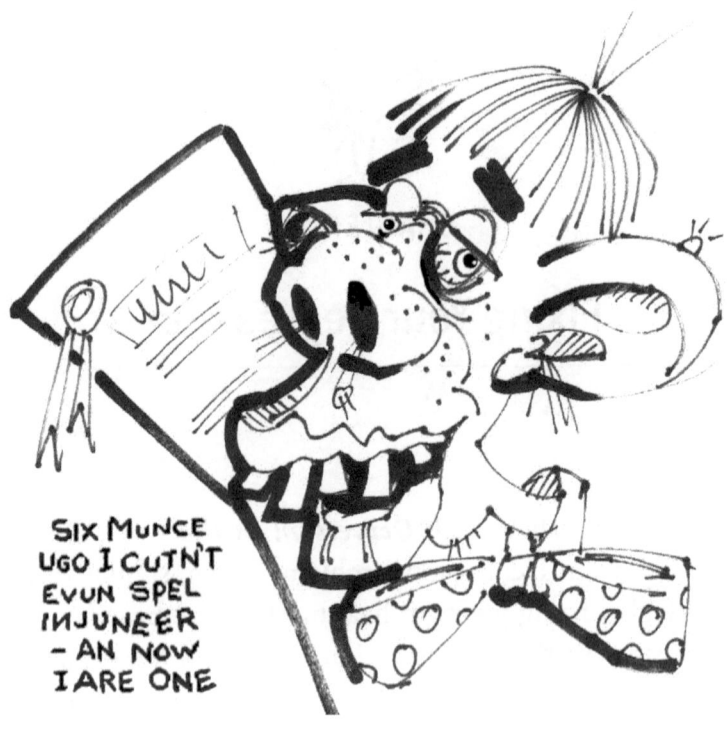

SIX MUNCE
UGO I CUTN'T
EVUN SPEL
INJUNEER
– AN NOW
I ARE ONE

you may have, but getting rid of Depression is the second thing you have to do in your life right now. Number one is to survive, but that is largely taken care of by your own body… THE ULTIMATE SURVIVAL MACHINE.

You are not guilty of Depression, you just have it and you want it gone, fast! You may have even done it to yourself but you didn't mean to. You probably look at the guy or girl next door and say, "you're a prick," or "I'm better than you are. I work harder, my kids are nicer, I have a better job and you drink too much. I don't deserve to have Depression." Well who cares? If you are depressed, it doesn't matter how diligent you are, how many school meetings you attend, how often you go to church, how much money you have, or whether you coach the kids' footy team. This disease does not discriminate. You possibly have no idea how, when, or why you got it. To a large extent, neither do I. I do know how to fix it though, and it's not hard and it doesn't take a lifetime of discipline or eating mung beans.

I have a bet with my wife a couple of times a week. We bet on all sorts of stuff. Our usual bet is one dollar. We bet on what time school drop-off will occur, whether I'll catch a fish, even what type of fish it will be. As soon as the bet is made, I do what I can to manipulate the odds in my favour. I might want to delay Monica, if the bet is that drop-off will be after 8.30am. The best way is to engage her in conversation or ask her to make me toast. Engaging her in conversation is easy, but getting her to make me toast is more of an advanced skill. I think I win just over half the time, which will do me.

I will bet you that I can fix your Depression in a month or at least make you feel a whole lot better. The bet is one dollar. If I lose, details of how to redeem your dollar are at the end of this chapter.

I won't ask you to sacrifice anything (much) or give up anything, or change your favourite thing; unless that thing is snorting cocaine daily or consuming burgers for every meal. Both of those things I consider crazy, but I don't judge you. I just say do it occasionally, if you have to.

All you have to do is open your mind to the possibility that maybe, on balance, I might be suggesting reasonable things that make some sense, and may help. I can't guarantee that you will live to 100. I can't guarantee you won't get cancer or get hit by a bus. I can't really guarantee anything except that I cured my Depression quickly and unexpectedly, I have seen others do it, and I reckon you can do it too.

So, let's get started.

Depression is not in your head. It's an illness just like measles or the flu or cancer. It has to do with what you put in and on your body. In other words, it's biological; a physical condition. Don't worry, I'm not telling you to go vegetarian or alcohol free or any other such nonsense. Your Depression has little to do with not getting a raise at work, or that the kids drive you crazy, or the fact that your father was an asshole. In other words, it's not caused by external circumstances. You will deal with those things in time, or not, and they could make your life worse for sure. Depression is caused by internal circumstances, like incorrect food choices and medicines and chemicals that you ingest or apply. The other things, difficulties in your life, may even be the trigger for Depression, but it's what you put in and on your body that makes Depression hang around.

Take my example; I have a great wife, a big house, three kids that don't drive me crazy all the time, and I had Depression. Jamie Packer, Australia's 10th richest man, had or has Depression. Robin Williams, the great comedian, had Depression. Winston Churchill also had Depression. Angelina Jolie and Michael Phelps allegedly had Depression. People with plenty of money, resources and great health care, still get Depression. Shit, do you think the Indians (you know from India) don't have poverty, lack of sanitation, child abuse, alcoholism, slavery, religious persecution, lack of opportunity? None of that stuff makes much difference as far as Depression goes. It seems to me that there are an awful lot of them (Indians I mean), try 1.2 billion. They are not going out of style. I have been to India and I can tell you they just suck it up and get on with life. I assume some of them get Depression too, but if you see the way many of them live, it's hard to believe that most of them don't suffer from Depression, but they don't.

I'm not telling you to suck it up and get on with life…that rarely solves the problem of Depression. That's what people who have never experienced Depression say to those who have it. They don't have a clue what Depression is like, but you know what I'm talking about!

I am just saying that Depression doesn't come from external sources. If it did, probably everyone would be depressed. We all have tragedies in our lives. Some are bigger and more constant than others. The thing is, we all feel those tragedies in our own context. Some really awful things happen in the world, no doubt, but the thing is, large numbers of people who suffer from Depression are just regular people like you and me. Others go through immense tragedy (like the entire Jewish race) with grief, but without lasting Depression. This is what led me to believe that

Depression is biological, not psychological.

Don't get me wrong, psychology and psychoanalysis has its place, a big place. The thing is; I hope to give you the best biological basis to solve your Depression. If you still need psychology, you'll work that out. I am not a good person to ask about that. What I am saying is that you can have all the psychology in the world, but if you don't solve the biology, Depression will most probably continue to be a problem for you. In my view, the notion that Depression is a psychological condition is largely wrong. I'm pretty sure that after you read this book, and apply these simple techniques, you will agree with me.

Dr Jordan Peterson is a world-famous clinical psychologist and a professor. He is brilliant and solves all sorts of problems, but he and his daughter suffered Depression for years. They didn't fix it until both changed their diets. Jordan and his daughter changed to the All-Meat diet, not only fixing their Depression but also many other health problems they were suffering. I have tried the All-Meat diet and it's brilliant. The reason this diet works is that quality meat provides all the essential vitamins, fats and proteins, and minerals (in the correct form) that a person needs. I am not going to write further about it in this book, but it does work. The point I am making, again, is that Depression comes from what you put in and on your body, and to some extent, what you don't put in and on your body. Our modern lifestyle is quite un-natural in many aspects and that loss of nature can cause illness and Depression.

The following pages contain my list of things that I believe will fix your Depression. I'm not sure if they're in order, but they could be.

Probiotics fix your gut health ☑

Probiotics (live bacteria) is how I solved my Depression. Prebiotics (food for bacteria) are important too. It's all about gut health. The other stuff (mentioned below) I learned about later. You don't have to take

Probiotics and Prebiotics forever. Not all probiotics are created equal. I will elaborate later in the book. There are bucket loads of science to back me up on this. Probiotics (bacteria) eat prebiotics (fibre). Most of us have spent much of our lives damaging our guts by taking antibiotics and just plain ignoring our gut health. It's understandable because the science behind the importance of gut health is relatively new.

Sunshine ☑

This is sun exposure, around midday, with no protection whatsoever; no sunscreen, sunglasses or glass or plastic covering your eyes. Aim for 20 minutes a day between 10am and 2pm. If you can't get sunshine then you have to eat sunshine. It's not hard to do. For example, eating fish is like eating sunshine. Cod liver oil is too, as is butter. Getting out in the sun for 20 minutes a day and exposing your skin and eyes to the sun (don't look directly at it) may not cure your Depression on its own, but it will make you feel a whole lot better. It's the vitamin D, in case you were wondering. NOTE: If you happen to die from skin cancer in the next few weeks after over-exposure to the sun, that I caused, then let me know and I will send you a card.

Salt ☑

Aim for two teaspoons a day of raw, unprocessed salt (10g/day). Space it out. More if you can get it. That is about double the recommended intake suggested by the WHO (World Health Organisation). I am not saying to do it forever, just for the next few months while you fix your Depression. My research tells me that you should do it forever, but you will make your own choice on that. NOTE: If you happen to die from hypertension/heart disease, or salt poisoning in the next few weeks, again, let me know and I will send you a card.

Water ☑

Drink when you're thirsty and not too much more. Aim for 1-2 litres per day. Make it rainwater when you can. Filter the water if you can't get rainwater. Add some lemon juice, it makes a difference. NOTE: Again, if death occurs from dehydration in the next few weeks, call me.

Avoid Poisons ☑

All medicines are, by definition, poisons. I'm not joking. Look it up. That doesn't mean you should never take medicine. Take it for a while then stop. If you need medicine, vitamins or supplements to fix your Depression then take them. If you are on an antidepressant then I admire your courage. It's way better to take antidepressants and stay alive than the alternative. They worked for me some of the time. The problem with antidepressants is that if you don't change the other things I mentioned above, then you're unlikely to be cured. Anti-depressants do not cure Depression but they do hold it at bay, usually. What I am saying here is to beware of all medicines and even vitamin supplements. Be informed. They absolutely all have side effects and occasionally the side effects can be Depression or other neurological disturbances.

In an article from the JAMA (Journal of American Medical Association), they state: *"In over 200 medicines commonly available, Depression is listed as one of the possible side effects. During the study period, more than one third of the US population were taking one or more of these medicines."*
(Web source:www.jamanetwork.com/journals/jama/fullarticle/2684607)

Medicines are not the only poisons out there. Many people, including myself, try to eat organic foods. People should try to limit or reduce traces of poisons in their diet. Chlorine is a poison and it's in the water that you drink every day. You can't eliminate all poisons, but you can attempt to reduce them.

Vitamins ☑

Vitamins are basically poisons, unless you obtain them in their natural form; that form being food sources. If you're taking a vitamin or prescribed one, by all means keep taking it, but be wary of vitamins or supplements. Like medicines, there can be side effects.

Minerals ☑

I readily admit to being very non-expert on this topic. If you live in a modern, wealthy country like Australia, USA, Germany or Singapore, and your diet is reasonable, your chances of being mineral deficient are low. On the other hand, it can happen, and rather easily too. I am just trying to give you the best biological method of solving the issue of Depression. My research tells me that the 'biggie' minerals for people with Depression are Iron, Sodium, Chloride (not Chlorine), Potassium, Iodine, Magnesium and Lithium. What I would say is to concentrate on the bigger issues (I mentioned above) and if you have a mineral deficiency, that is the last thing on my list that you need to address. Hopefully you will have fixed your Depression well before mineral deficiencies come into play.

Hey, you don't have to believe me, or do all the things I suggest, or any of them. But if I'm right (and I believe I am) then it will cost you virtually nothing, you will see results quickly, and as I see it, there is no downside. I mean you might get skin cancer, heart disease, dehydration or a tummy upset, 20 years from now… still, fix your Depression first and worry about that other stuff later. Worry about living to 100 later. So that's the basics: Get sunshine, eat more salt, drink enough good water, take probiotics and avoid poisons. It's pretty simple really. If you're interested, in the following pages I'll tell you the 'why'.

Out of Africa

While I was writing this book, a friend of mine told me a story. It almost summarises exactly what I just stated about salt, minerals, and probiotics, if not sunshine.

There is a medicine man in Africa who is apparently having success in curing Depression, literally overnight.

What you do is arrive in his village then the tribe kills a sheep. You drink the blood from the animal, eat the meat, and then they make a blanket out of the sheep's stomach in which you sleep. Apparently, you wake up the next day, if indeed you slept at all, and your Depression is gone.

When my friend told me this story, I said, "of course that would work." I didn't mean that arrogantly, it just made sense to me.

You get the salt and minerals from the blood and eating the meat. You get vitamin D (processed sunshine) from the meat as well. The sheep's stomach is loaded with beneficial bacteria (probiotics) that get into your system by breathing them in, through your skin, or by ingestion. The bacteria from a 'natural sheep' are superior to probiotics they manufacture in a laboratory. Wild bacteria are more diverse and less fragile than lab/factory produced probiotics.

I mean you could sleep in a sheep's stomach in Australia if you wanted to, but I'm not sure how long it would take for that therapy to gain TGA (Therapeutic Goods Association) approval.

If you don't have time to go to Africa and sleep in a sheep's stomach, then I suggest you try the ideas in this book. It's sort of the same, without the 'ickyness' factor.

Just Try It!

There are some ideas in this book that I'm just going to ask you to believe, because I have tried them, and I have done research as to why they work. I don't necessarily have hard evidence that would stand up in a court of law, but I have done my research. What I want you to do is just give it a try for a while, not forever, unless it sounds crazy or dangerous, which I don't believe any of the concepts are. I would also encourage you to do your own research, but you have to drill down and smartly research. If, for example, you do an internet search on salt consumption and health, the first ten or fifty sites will warn you against higher salt consumption. You need to balance your research. You have to read articles that support your view or the mainstream view, and you have to read the opposing view as well (or you can just let me do it). For further example, research SALT, health good or bad? You may get a balance of arguments. It's the same with sunshine. But do you have the motivation to do such research? Do you have the time to do it? It takes shitloads of time. I had that time, and the interest, so I did the research. And don't believe everything the mainstream tells you. Don't believe everything I tell you either…try it for yourself, or research it for yourself, experiment for yourself. In the next chapter I'll introduce you to myself, and my family. As you can see from this recent photograph, we are just like you.

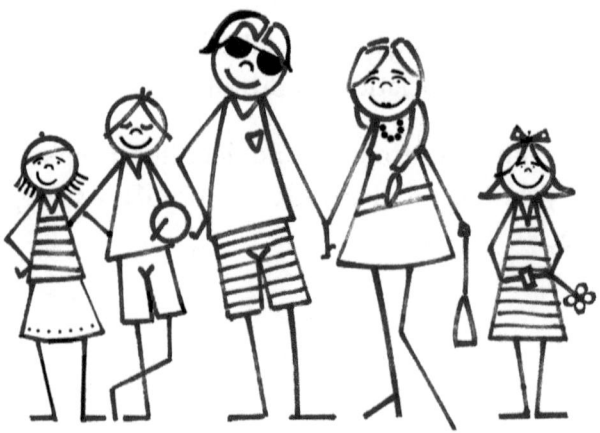

P.S. The American Plan

Just in case this book ever reaches the shores of America...

This book is NOT written on the American Plan.

Don't get me wrong, I love Americans and have visited the country many times, I even worked there for a while and have American friends. But when it comes to selling a thing, or an idea, can you Americans just get to the point?

I don't want to wade through a 45-minute video presentation to find the answer in the last 5 minutes. I don't want to read a 200-page book and have the answer delivered in the last chapter. I want to know the answer now! I want to know how much that miracle gadget costs now! I don't want to know all the extras I'll get, and I don't want to be upsized. I just want the answer now!

So here is my prescription for getting rid of Depression, now!

- **Get some probiotics/fix your gut**
- **Get more sunshine**
- **Eat more salt**
- **Drink quality water, but not too much**
- **Stop taking poisons**

The reasons why this prescription works are found in later chapters of this book.

So I've given you the answers, now! Next, we can deal with the detail. If you don't like the answers, you are free to look for yourself. I know this works because I've done it myself.

While I'm on it Americans, I have used the metric system and the English words mostly in place of American equivalents. This will not make it difficult for you. Here are some examples:

Arse	=	Ass. Basically I'm referring to your butt, or bottom in Australian
mg	=	milligrams as in vitamin measurements. Same in American English
Tonne	=	Ton or 1000Kgs, or 2000 pounds
Kilogram	=	Kg or 2.2 lbs
Grams	=	g. 30 grams equals one ounce, except when you are buying Marijuana. They only give you 20g. Who would have thought that drug dealers were scammers?
Fibre	=	fiber, the roughage stuff in vegetables
Poo	=	shit, faeces or feces. 'Shit' in any language
Fuck	=	an expression, adjective, adverb or noun and sometimes a verb, in fact, probably the most versatile word in the English language. I'm sure when you see it, you'll get my drift. I believe it has approximately the same meaning in all dialects of English, Russian, German, and Japanese.

P.P.S.

My inspiration to write this book came from another book I read (it's American) called *The Subtle Art of Not Giving a F*ck*. That's how I came up with this plain green cover and deliberately placed swear words on the front…it gets your attention.

How to redeem your dollar in the unlikely event that I lose the bet

Send me a short letter, no more than ten pages, and no fewer than five, stating which of the methods I described and how long you tried each one. Don't give me too much praise or it will go to my head. Oh, and naturally I'll need the original receipt, a short description of the bookseller, and what they were wearing that day.

You can post it on my facebook page '**blackdogtoolbox**'. Please include your name, rank and serial number, so I can send your dollar. Specify your preferred currency, otherwise it will be in Zimbabwean dollars.

In fact, I'm so confident that my ideas will help you, I am prepared to give odds. Let's say 2:1.

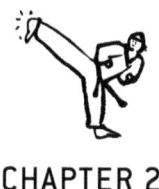

CHAPTER 2

Qualifications: About Me

This book is approximately 50% my experiences and anecdotal evidence, and 50% science and evidence-based studies. I don't want to dwell on the issue of my qualifications, but I would like to give you some confidence that I have a vague idea of what I'm talking about.

My basic premise is that the answers to solving Depression are found in chemistry, biology, history and evolution; important things that can't be ignored. I would like to say the stronger forces are chemistry/biology but that is based on our evolutionary history anyway, so they are all intertwined.

My most important qualification as far as you are concerned is that I had Depression and I solved it. I suffered from it for a bit over 2 years from April 2011 to June 2013. I suspect I had bouts of it during my life that were more fleeting, or I simply didn't recognise, but in 2011 it was pretty sustained.

I have a degree in Engineering as I mentioned, which is just a glorified train driver, but my wife has a PhD in Microbiology. No one knows what Microbiology is, but let's call it Biochemistry. Microbiologists actually study bacteria and tiny living things. Her father had a DSc in Microbiology, which is the next level above a PhD. (You don't get to become a DSc, unless you're invited by the other geniuses). My wife's mother was a science teacher. My father was an industrial chemist. One of my daughters is studying Pharmacy and the other is studying Biochemical Engineering, so you could say that chemistry and biology run pretty strongly in the family. If my son doesn't study science or engineering, I will be surprised. I just hope it's not the science of gaming!

I'm not a doctor or psychologist, which I'm pretty happy about, because I don't have to comply with all the professional standards and other restrictions on their methods. I can say pretty much what I want, and I try to practice what I preach, but being a human, I often fall short.

My two best qualifications though, are that I had Depression, and I cured it. I'm just like you, even though we don't know each other. My digestive system is just like yours. My heart and organs are approximately in the same place as yours. My blood has the same acidity as yours, I want to live a long and happy life, I want the same things for my children. I want peace and harmony and excitement and clean water and a nice house and security and warmth and respect, just like you. People today carry on about diversity, but maybe, it's the sameness about us all that is more important. The point I'm trying to make is that I am just like you and I don't even know you. We have much more in common than things that divide us. We even share about 90%+ of the same genes.

On the other hand, I'm probably better at chemistry than you. And perhaps better at using the internet to solve problems, and way better at uniting chemistry and history with evolution than you. I truly hope that what I write here will help you or your friend fix a big problem. I was 100% successful with myself. I've also been very successful with other people I have helped using these methods. It may not help you, but it won't harm you either.

I would like to make money from this book. Hey, I like money as much as the next guy. But if I don't, it won't bother me. I have enough. At this stage I don't have a supplement to sell, but I may have in the future, I don't know yet. I do have a website which contains much of the information here and more besides. I'm happy for you to go there, but if you read this and it gives you what you want, then you don't really need to.

My website is: **blackdogtoolbox.com.au**

About Me

I'm pretty much a regular person like you.

I love my wife and she loves me. That's a big help with Depression, but it doesn't stop you from getting it. My kids are good performers at school and happy most of the time. Our family has taken a holiday to New Zealand or North America or Europe every year for about ten years, so we are not short of dough. That helps too, but again, it doesn't stop you from suffering Depression.

I live near the beach and go surfing, windsurfing, or kitesurfing every other day in summer (the season lasts about 9 months in Queensland where I live). I play tennis at least once a week and go to the gym once a week. I eat a pretty good diet (not perfect, but plenty of organics and fresh meat). I drink too much wine, but I try to stick with organic when I can.

Reading the above, how could I have had Depression? Life was pretty good.

Well, there was a trigger (there almost always is).

In January 2011 South East Queensland was hit with a big flood that caused significant damage to a property I owned. The property was my main source of income, and I had a hefty mortgage. This caused me a lot of anxiety and the Depression followed soon after.

The anxiety and the disaster (flood) turned out to be less of a problem than anticipated, but the Depression stayed. I feel that the Depression would likely have come anyway, eventually, but this event accelerated the process. I think this often happens with many people. Depression is possibly lurking then BANG…a big life event pushes you over the edge.

I continued my sports and exercising, right through the Depression years. I spent time outdoors and got plenty of sunlight, I worked with my hands and also my head. Nothing helped. I spent huge amounts of time researching natural cures. I spent plenty of money on vitamins and supplements that are supposed to help with Depression, e.g. Vitamin D, vitamin B12, magnesium, amino acids, fish oil, herbs and some pretty exotic stuff and combinations. I went to a health farm for 10 days. I went on a 3-day retreat performing yoga for the first time and eating the Ayurveda way. I learned a lot. Nothing really helped, although there were some fleeting improvements. I tried some antidepressants; they worked okay too.

Of course, I dabbled with meditation, read about mindfulness, thought about religion, my personality, and my past mistakes, but I really felt the answers were biological rather than situational, which turned out to be true.

One thing I should say is that I am very responsive to medicines and supplements. If they work for me, I usually know straight away. If there is a side effect, I usually get it (even if I don't know that there are side effects before I take it). If there is a placebo effect, it never seems to work on me. Doesn't matter how positive I am about something, if it doesn't work, it just doesn't work. Consequently, the things that do work come as a complete surprise to me because I am not expecting a result. Maybe it's a reverse placebo effect; who knows?

I guess this may be the result of being particularly self-aware. Maybe some people think that's conceited, I hope not, it's not meant to be. I just take notice of those little changes that go on around me and in me. I then look for the reason why. Maybe it's the way I've been taught as an engineer; I don't know. I am not telling you to do this, I'm just telling you that I solved my Depression. I'm pretty sure I can solve yours too, and I know why.

If my qualifications aren't enough, I forgive you for being sceptical.

What I suggest is that Depression can be explained at least as much by basic biology as by psychology. Don't believe me? Go and get yourself tested for the following: check your salt levels, check your iron levels, check your vitamin D levels (sunshine), check your vitamin B12 levels, and if you're not having regular, daily, well-formed bowel movements, get your gut checked (maybe a colonoscopy, maybe a stool sample test). If you are in Australia, most of those tests are free. Hey, maybe solving those issues doesn't fix your Depression, but it will improve your general health anyway, and that can't be bad. Don't ignore the basics of your physical health, it may well be strongly related to your mental health.

Here's a quote I found by accident some months after I wrote the above part about getting tested:

> "In January 2015, an international collaboration on the topic was published in *The Lancet Psychiatry*, stating that mounting evidence indicates vital relationships between diet quality and mental health."

Evidence is so compelling, they say, that psychiatry and public health should recognise and embrace nutrition as a key component of mental health.

> "Studies have demonstrated that omega-3s, B vitamins - especially folate and B12 – choline, iron, zinc, magnesium, S-adenosyl methionine (SAMe), vitamin D and amino acids are linked to brain health," the researchers remarked.

> "While we advocate for these to be consumed in the diet where possible, additional select prescription of these as nutraceuticals

– nutrient supplements – may also be justified," stated lead author Dr Jerome Sarris from *AFP Relaxnews.*

(Web source: www.thestar.com.my/lifestyle/health/2015/06/17/fermented-food-like-tempeh-can-make-you-more-sociable)

The Lancet is an extremely well regarded scientific journal.

Oh, one more thing, I am very non-conformist. If everyone is doing one thing, I always look for the alternative view and give that a try too. It doesn't always work, but it's often worth a try. Lots of people try a vegetarian or vegan diet these days. Fair enough, I have tried vegetarianism myself. The point is though, it's just an experiment. The All-Meat diet I mentioned in Chapter 1 is an experiment too and it has plenty of scientific and historical backing to show that it works as far as general nutrition goes. I found it very beneficial. Unless you try both experiments (all vegetables or all meat), you can't possibly know what the correct result is for you. I know many people become vegetarians for ethical reasons, like saving the planet or animal cruelty etc. Again, fair enough, not that they have any idea whether that helps or not. If you suffer from Depression, forget all of that stuff, forget ethics, forget saving the planet, forget trying to live to 100. **The best thing you can do for yourself and your family, and the planet, is to fix your Depression. Save the planet later.**

In regard to the swearing that you'll encounter in this book: I've tried to convey this story in the same way that people talk to each other, you know, as a conversation. That almost always involves swearing. I have attempted not to overuse it though.

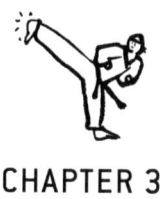

CHAPTER 3

My Lists

From Chapter 1 you'll recall my list: Sunshine, salt, water, and probiotics; my top things to help cure Depression.

In this chapter, I describe the causes of Depression and the small changes you can make to your lifestyle to alleviate it.

My Top 6 Causes of Depression

These are not the only causes of Depression and anxiety, but they are also causes of poor gut health. They appear in approximate order of importance.

You may find this a bit overwhelming but there are simple ways to minimise the damage that I'm about to describe.

1. Difficult life events/stress. Stress is a by-product of being alive. It's obviously possible to reduce stress, but you can't eliminate it. If you gave away your worldly possessions then you would have the stress of acquiring worldly possessions. There is always the stress of having enough in the future. Stress will never leave you. Major stress though, is often the start of Depression. Absolutely everyone will suffer major stress at some stage in life. Not everyone will suffer Depression though (fortunately).

2. The modern food supply is littered with problems.

3. The modern lifestyle/cleanliness/loss of nature. Lack of sunshine is an obvious example of No.3.

4. Chemically treated water. Again, virtually unavoidable and way better than contaminated water.

5. Antibiotics*

6. Prescription drugs**

<u>Note:</u> *I don't advise anyone to stop taking antibiotics now, or in the future. **I don't advise anyone to stop taking any drug prescribed by a doctor.

Depression may have occurred in the past, before modernity, though Depression seems to be in epidemic proportions today.

I came across this list at *Phion.com.au,* an Australian manufacturer of health supplements and water purification technology. I just couldn't believe the similarity with my list, so I thought I'd share it! I can assure you that I have no interest in this company, and at the time of writing, I've not tried their products. This is pure coincidence only. I am talking about Depression, whereas they are referring to gut health, but to my mind, they are one and the same.

> *"The Top 7 Gut Biology balance and immune system destroyers include:*
>
> *1. Prescription antibiotics*
>
> *2. Sugar*
>
> *3. Tap water (positive charge)*
>
> *4. GMO foods (most processed food-based corn and soy)*
>
> *5. Grains (not activated, i.e. soaked overnight or fermented)*
>
> *6. Emotional stress (e.g. grief, anger, resentment, etc.)*
> *Love, joy and hope have healthy effects on gut biology balance*
>
> *7. Chemicals in processed food and pharmaceutical medications."*

Here's a list of my 'Top Things to Avoid' to help cure your Depression

Keep in mind that I'm suggesting 'avoid', not necessarily delete.

AVOID	BETTER CHOICES
White Rice	Brown rice
Simple starches	Prebiotic Fibre
Canola Oil/cheap oil	Olive oil/animal fats
Margarine	Butter
Paracetamol	Aspirin/Ibuprofen
Cheap or cask wine	Bottled wine (decent quality)
Grain-fed meat	Grass-fed meat
Diet drinks	Sugary drinks
Sugary drinks	Water
Tap water	Filtered water or rainwater
Sugar substitutes	Sugar or honey
Fruit Juice	Fruit
Low fat milk	High fat milk
Sunscreen	Exposure to UV light
Cheap beer	German or quality beer
Antibacterial soap/toothpaste	Un-medicated cosmetics
Food with no value	Live food/fermented food
Social Media	Reading books
Veganism	Meat, Fish, animal products
Fast food	Traditional food
Supplements	Traditional food
Screen Time	Natural environments

This might sound like just a regular laundry list of health recommendations, but I can assure you it's not. This is all about recovering your mental health quickly, without upending your lifestyle.

Before I leave here, I'm going to give the briefest possible reasons for the above list, based on the science I have learned whilst writing the book, and my own experience.

Rice

White rice for the masses (you and me) has only existed for about 150 years. Before that it was all brown rice. Brown rice contains fibre - prebiotics (you will read about this later). Fibre feeds bacteria that live in your gut and help to produce healthy brain chemicals.

Simple starches are in the same category as white rice. I know it's hard to believe, but white rice and simple starches are really sugar in disguise, it's not my view, it's a scientific fact. By the way, when I was a kid, brown rice sucked. There were always grains that were hard as rocks. Whatever they do with it today, it has vastly improved.

Canola Oil

Canola oil was only invented in the last 50 years. We have no idea where this experiment will lead. Olive oil has been around for thousands of years. Have that instead. It costs more but it's worth it.

Margarine vs Butter

I could say see above, but that's too easy. Stick some margarine out in the garage and some butter. The ants, flies and your dog will eat the butter. I'm not so sure about the margarine. Butter is natural. Margarine doesn't exist without major human intervention. Butter has existed for thousands of years. Margarine is less than 200 years old.

Paracetamol vs Aspirin

Even though aspirin is synthetic, it's based on willow bark that's been around for thousands of years. Paracetamol is a wholly new substance. The paracetamol is processed by your liver and is at least as damaging as alcohol; worse in my opinion. Aspirin works and has far more evidence-based benefits. There's a rare syndrome that stops people from taking Aspirin. It's so rare as to be negligible, and the evidence is not strong.

Wine

It's the preservatives basically, that make wine unhealthy. I mean there is more to it, but not much. Wine is about as natural a product as you can get. Cheap wine is often loaded with chemicals. Some expensive wines are too. The price point is just a rule of thumb. Wine is otherwise a very natural product. Cheap wines often use oak shavings to give the oakiness flavour. Oak actually contains tiny amounts of poison. That's why aged barrels are more prized than new barrels. Most of the poison has been removed by the original process.

Grain-fed Meat

Animals don't eat grain unless they are starving. Animals (and humans) should eat what they are designed to eat. Animals fed grain have a wholly different fat profile than grass-fed animals. Meat animals should eat grass. It's complex but important.

Sugar Substitutes

Anything produced using modern processing methods is suspect. Not necessarily bad for you, but we just don't know yet. Beware of anything that your great-grandparents wouldn't have eaten. Sugar has been around for hundreds of years. Sugar substitutes are new and we just don't yet know if they are good for us.

Fruit Juice

Concentrating things has the tendency to ruin it. Pluck an orange from the tree and eat it. That's the best way.

Low Fat Milk

The same principle applies as stated above. Once you start mucking about with nature, the chances are you might not get it right. Nature has been around for a long time and tends to get things right. Low fat milk is not just regular milk with some fat removed. Low fat milk is thoroughly tampered with. Did you know this? Fat reduced milk has a higher sugar content (lactose) than regular milk.

Sunscreen

Again, the above rules apply. Sunscreen may be natural, but the chemicals are concentrated. The sun has been shining for billions of years. If it were a killer, as it's made out to be, then we wouldn't even be here. Let some of it into your life and onto your skin.

Beer

Germany has the best beer in the world, by a country mile. The laws relating to how beer can be produced in Germany date back 500 years. By law, German beer is completely natural. Regardless what kind of beer you drink, observe how it makes you feel health wise and gut wise. It's very easy to become loyal to a brand for no good reason. There are many health problems associated with alcoholic beverages but the truth is; many of them aren't caused by the alcohol itself, but by other factors in the drink. For example, you cry in your Gin because of the quinine in the tonic water, not because of the alcohol in the Gin.

Antibacterial Cosmetics

Antibacterial chemicals kill good and bad bacteria. Many bacteria are helpful. This is discussed in detail in the following chapters.

Live Food

Live food is full of beneficial bacteria and pre-digested to unlock the nutrients for you.

Social Media/Screen Time vs Nature

There is more to this than just my personal views. There is science to back this. Screens, especially close up screens, produce blue light that sends confusing signals to your brain.

Fast Food

Well I would have thought this was obvious...

Supplements

I just suggest getting your vitamins, minerals and nutrients from real food, rather than concentrates and laboratory-made substances. Let me clarify this because sometimes the damage done to your body and gut by modern life, needs extra firepower to overcome it.

Sure... it would be great if we could all just wander off into the bush and eat a traditional diet, living off the land and avoiding modernity, but we can't, so sometimes, artificial supplements can help. It just pays to embrace nature and avoid artificial things if you can, that's all. I'd rather you eat an orange any day, over taking a vitamin C tablet.

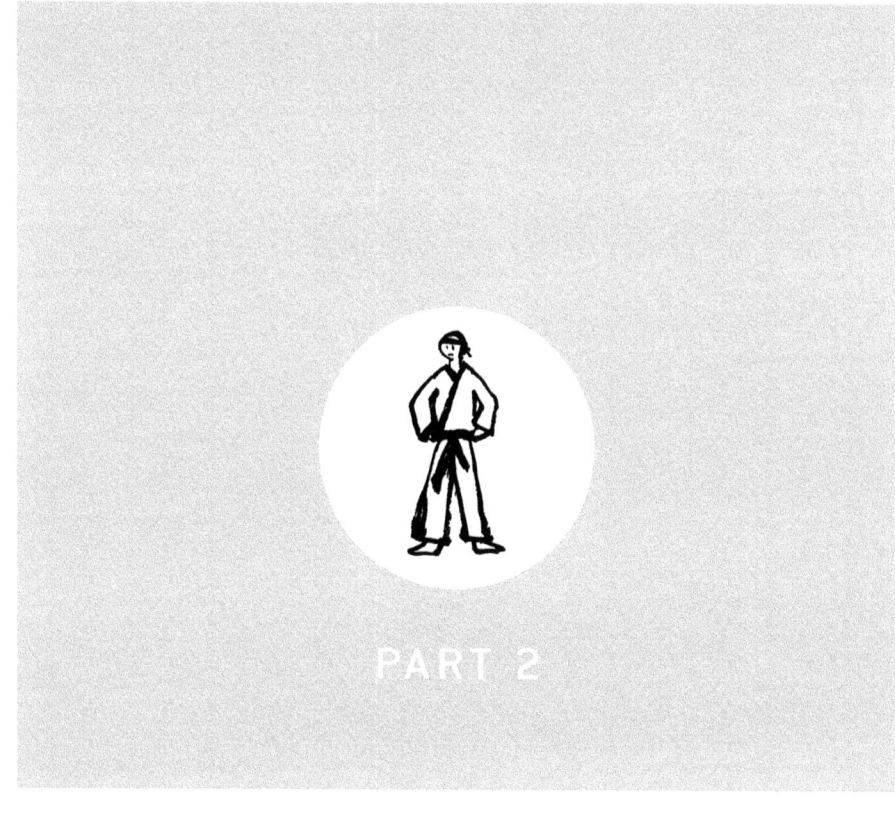

PART 2

SOME OF THE SCIENCE
BEHIND DEPRESSION

CHAPTER 4

Theories of Depression

What is Depression?

This will be the shortest section of the book. All I know is what it felt like to me. I don't know how it feels to you or anyone else you know. My contention is that if you are suffering from Depression you know it, unless you're a child and don't know what's going on. Your body 'seems' to be functioning normally, but you know 'in your head' that something is not right. You know what happiness or normality is like, and this is not it, this is different.

I think if I try and put words in your head about what I think Depression is, then that has as much chance of harming you, as helping you. You don't need the additional burden of how it felt to me. I'd just like to say hang in there, because there is a way out. You can fix this and it may not be as hard or as long as you think. If you want to know what Depression 'feels like' you can look it up on the internet.

P. S.

And don't confuse Depression with sadness and regret. Sadness and regret are normal human emotions. When I had Depression for example, I could be out on a tennis court, playing well and even winning, and still be depressed. Depression is a biological condition, an illness if you like.

Types of Depression

As I understand it, there's more than one kind of Depression, for example: PTSD (Post Traumatic Stress Disorder), Bipolar, Post-natal Depression, Psychosis and Schizophrenia. Let us say that in this book we are talking about your regular 'garden variety' (unipolar) Depression. I'm confident that my methods would be helpful for all types of Depression, but I just don't know enough about the other types. There are certainly studies indicating that probiotics can be useful for PTSD and Post-natal Depression cases, and that the gut bacteria of these sufferers differ from people without these conditions.

It's funny how we treat Depression differently to almost all other diseases.

Take Scurvy for example; we know it's caused by a lack of fresh food and vitamin C. If you have Thyroid disease, we know it's related to Iodine metabolism. A bacterial infection; you've contracted some bad bacteria and there are antibiotics to combat it. If you have Osteoporosis, it's from a lack of calcium. If you have Diabetes (Type 2), it's from too much sugar.

Is it so hard to believe then that when you suffer from Depression, there is a chemical or biological basis to it?

So, if a guy goes to the doctor with Scurvy (pretty rare today), the doctor gives him a vitamin C tablet; a bacterial infection, an antibiotic; diabetes, well stop eating sugar for starters. In other words, we give something or take something away.

Now apart from antidepressants, most depressed people will receive some kind of counselling, but you don't get counselled when you have a bacterial infection, or Scurvy, or Diabetes. Somehow, it's your behaviour or your attitude to life, or your upbringing, or your lack of religious belief that causes your Depression.

Well it's my contention that with Depression, it's the same as with these other ailments. There is something missing, or too much of, in your diet or your lifestyle. It's not something that will be fixed by counselling. Hey, I'm not against counselling, but I am saying that Depression is caused by an overabundance, or lack of something, and I believe I know what the main culprit is. It's something called serotonin, and serotonin is created by your gut bacteria, which you've been ignoring for years. Read on and find out.

Serotonin Theory

Serotonin is a chemical messenger in your body, in a class of chemicals called neurotransmitters. They send signals around your body.

There are 13 neurotransmitters identified so far and probably more to come. Most of you will be familiar with some of the important ones listed here:

- Norepinephrine/epinephrine (most people call this adrenaline)
- Dopamine
- Serotonin
- GABA (Gamma Amino Butyric Acid)
- Acetylcholine
- Histamine

Below is a quote from the *Queensland Brain Institute* website:

"Key Neurotransmitters:

The first neurotransmitter to be discovered was a small molecule called acetylcholine. It plays a major role in the peripheral nervous system, where it is released by motor neurons and neurons of the autonomic nervous system. It also plays an important role in the central nervous system in maintaining cognitive function. Damage to the cholinergic neurons of the CNS is associated with Alzheimer disease.

Glutamate is the primary excitatory transmitter in the central nervous system. Conversely, a major inhibitory transmitter is its derivative γ-aminobutyric acid (GABA), while another inhibitory neurotransmitter is the amino acid called glycine, which is mainly found in the spinal cord.

Many neuromodulators, such as dopamine, are monoamines. There are several dopamine pathways in the brain, and this neurotransmitter is involved in many functions, including motor control, reward and reinforcement, and motivation.

Noradrenaline (or norepinephrine) is another monoamine, and is the primary neurotransmitter in the sympathetic nervous system where it works on the activity of various organs in the body to control blood pressure, heart rate, liver function and many other functions.

Neurons that use serotonin (another monoamine) project to various parts of the nervous system. As a result, serotonin is involved in functions such as sleep, memory, appetite, mood and others. It is also produced in the gastrointestinal tract in response to food.

Histamine, the last of the major monoamines, plays a role in metabolism, temperature control, regulating various hormones, and controlling the sleep-wake cycle, amongst other functions."

(Web source: https://qbi.uq.edu.au/brain/brain-physiology/what-are-neurotransmitters)

The important thing to know is that messages are sent around the body and to the brain by these chemicals/neurotransmitters.

The Serotonin Theory of Depression is the most widely understood and supported by most psychiatrists. The signals that serotonin sends are good signals, happy signals, like 'everything is okay, I'm awake and alert and everything is going alright.'

When you report symptoms of Depression to your doctor, the most frequent response will be to offer you a drug. The most widely prescribed class of drug (today) for Depression is an SSRI drug, and it's going to get its own heading:

Selective Serotonin Re Uptake Inhibitor (SSRI)

An SSRI Selects Serotonin (SS), meaning of all the neurotransmitters (there are at least 13), serotonin is the target. (R) Re-uptake is how serotonin moves in the synapse (nerve gap). The serotonin goes forward, and then a little bit goes backward (otherwise called re-uptake). The (I) is for Inhibitor, because it stops or slows the serotonin from going backwards. It's a bit complex so I use the term SSRI to mean a Serotonin Recycler. The most commonly used SSRI drugs are Zoloft, Prozac, Pristiq, and Celexa. Strictly speaking, Pristiq is an SNRI but let's not complicate things.

The SSRI drug makes better use of the serotonin you do have, which is not enough. The SSRI drug does not make more serotonin. I believe what you need to do is make more serotonin.

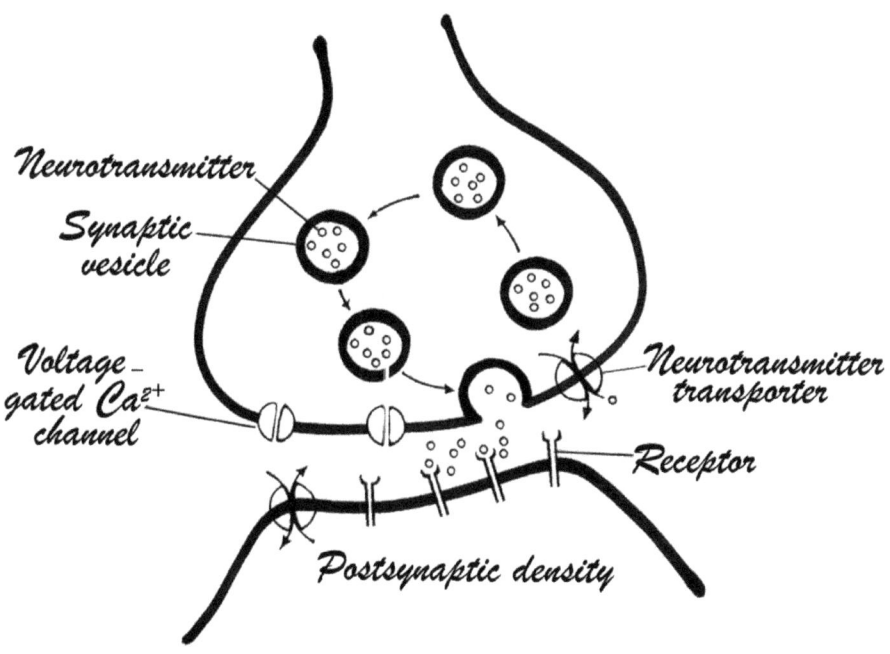

How to make Serotonin

Well how do you do that? There are a couple of really simple ways via food sources. For example, turkey, pork, chicken, and duck have loads of tryptophan, which is an amino acid (protein) that helps make serotonin. Real pasture-fed chicken has tryptophan, but real 'old-breed' pasture-fed chicken is hard to find today. Real parmesan cheese is also good. (I don't mean that powdered stuff in a can, but the real, fresh stuff from Italy). There are heaps of other serotonin foods and you don't need me to tell you all of them, look them up on the internet. You are looking for foods that contain TRYPTOPHAN. The thing about amino acids/ proteins is that modern farming techniques have a habit of changing them slightly, so they don't work as well. That's why turkey works better than chicken, because turkeys tend to have a more traditional diet than modern chickens. Chickens are supposed to eat grass and grasshoppers and bugs and worms, not wheat and corn. Sorry, I'm getting off topic. There is a guy called Dr Gundry who has this saying: *"You are what you eat, but you are also what you eat, eats"*.

That means if you eat a steak, you want that cow to have eaten grass (traditional cow diet) not grain, which is a non-traditional diet. If you are a vegetarian (and I hope you aren't) then you are eating a plant that extracts nutrients from soil. You want the soil to be good quality soil. If your plant eats poor soil, then it will have less nutritional value. As usual I digress.

To tell you the truth, the serotonin producing foods do work to some extent, but they are not the real action. The real action is getting your gut bacteria to make serotonin for you. We will get to that later.

Back to SSRI Drugs

The SSRI drugs can be effective but they do have side effects and change your metabolism. They slow your metabolism. Many of the SSRI drugs cause weight gain, but if they fix your Depression you probably don't care, at least until the weight becomes a problem. The SSRI drugs also take a few weeks to 'kick in'. I'm not against psychiatric drugs. If you think you need them, get them by all means. You need to know though, if you want to fix the actual cause of Depression, which is low serotonin, then there is more work to do. If you take, or are taking an SSRI drug, be aware that if you decide to cease its use, it takes a while, and that process needs to be managed.

What I'm trying to say, badly, is that if you are on an antidepressant, and you manage to cure your Depression, by it, my methods, or any other method, do not, then stop your antidepressant. These drugs have 'withdrawal sequalae'. In other words, withdrawal takes some effort and management, and you can get into trouble if you just stop 'cold turkey', whether you're 'cured' from Depression or not.

There are other important neurotransmitters, in particular GABA, Dopamine, and Noradrenaline (or Adrenalin if you like). GABA is for anti-anxiety or calming, Dopamine increases motivation and reward, and Noradrenaline is for energy and action.

You can take GABA supplements but they seem to have a very low efficacy. Interestingly, GABA supplements are produced through a fermentation process. Fermentation is what occurs in your gut… more on that later. Dopamine supplements are mildly effective but I don't know about their extended use or side effects. When you smoke a cigarette or take heroin, you get a Dopamine hit. That's why those things are so addictive. People love Dopamine. Dopamine is what you get when you jump out of a perfectly good aeroplane or bungy jump off a perfectly good bridge.

Benzodiazepines (eg. Valium, Clonazepam) work on the GABA system. Benzos are very helpful for anxiety, which is closely related to Depression. People with Depression often report anxiety as well. Benzos are considered highly addictive after only a month of use (more a dependency rather than an addiction). If you need them, they can be very helpful, especially if you only use them occasionally. Benzos work on the GABA system, they calm you down, but it's synthetic and ends up shrinking the GABA receptors. This is bad news. If you get addicted to Benzos and want to get off them, be very careful. I found myself addicted to them and weaning off was a very difficult experience. I've been told it's harder than kicking heroin. I wouldn't know, I've only tried Benzos, not heroin.

Back to the SSRI drugs... so they don't manufacture more serotonin or any other neurotransmitter. Benzos don't make more GABA. Dopamine supplements may make more Dopamine, but it's pretty ineffective.

About 80 to 90% of the serotonin in your body is found in your gut and is produced in your gut. By the gut, I'm referring to the large intestine/colon (i.e. the pipe that ends where the poo comes out). When you experience Depression/anxiety you can often have trouble sleeping. This is most likely due to low MELATONIN. Melatonin is the sleep hormone/neurotransmitter. Melatonin is made from serotonin. Not enough serotonin = not enough melatonin. So, you're exhausted but still can't sleep! Double whammy!

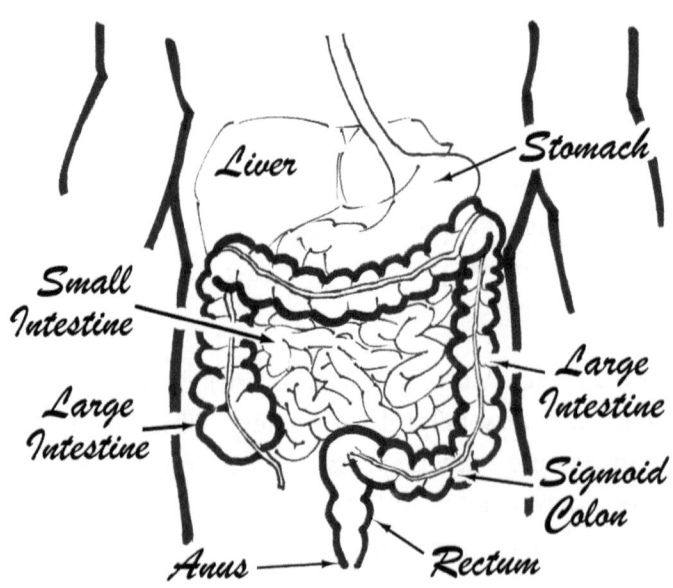

I have a theory that GABA, Dopamine and Noradrenaline are also manufactured in the gut; more about that later.

Sticking with serotonin, being the main action here…90% of your serotonin is found in your gut (you can look it up on the internet). I know almost everyone will say, "but Depression is in my head", or, "it feels like it's in my head." Well it isn't…it's in your GUT. That's your colon/large intestine as per the diagram opposite.

But assuming that concept is too hard, and I agree it's confronting, then let's assume that Depression is 'in your head' and it's caused by a lack of serotonin. If 90% of serotonin is in your gut, how does it get to your head?

Well, inside your body is a large nerve called the vagus nerve, a 'wandering' nerve (you know, from the word 'vague'). The vagus nerve is like a tree with many branches that connect every organ with every other organ. Signals travel along the branches of this tree. Many signals are serotonin signals.

By far the biggest branch of this tree, the TRUNK, is the superhighway that connects your gut to your brain. So, when the traffic gets cut off between your gut and your brain, you feel depressed. The traffic is the serotonin. That's the Serotonin Theory of Depression and pretty much all psychiatrists agree with it. They just express it differently, that's all. Serotonin is like the sap of the tree.

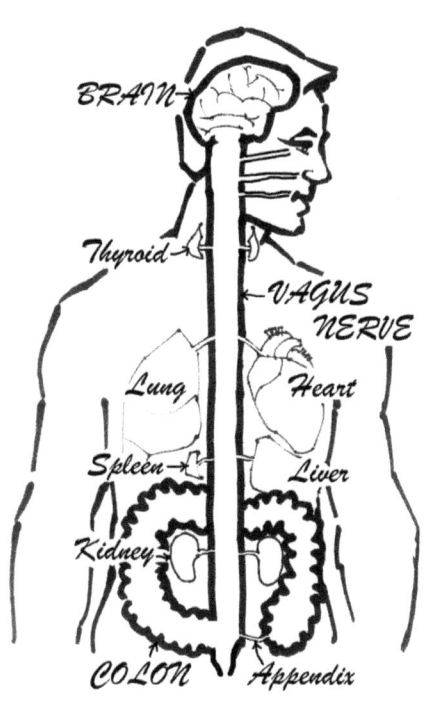

Depression is caused, primarily, by lack of serotonin. Where I don't agree with psychiatrists, is what to do about it. Having said that, I do agree that SSRI drugs work to some extent. My theory is that you need to make more serotonin from food or in your gut. I have done it myself, so I know it works. In the following chapters I aim to deliver information on how to improve your serotonin production, which hopefully will give you relief from Depression.

There are plenty of other theories about Depression and a growing movement against the Serotonin Theory. I admit, it may ultimately be replaced by something else that's likely to be a far more complex interaction of chemicals and neurotransmission…and beyond the comprehension of mere mortals like us. So let's just stick with the current model. It doesn't bother me too much what ultimately turns out to be true, because I know what worked for me, and many others. The theory of why it works could well be wrong, but the cure still requires fixing your gut bacteria and your diet.

P.S.

My research leads me to believe that the amount of serotonin you have, may not be the whole picture. There is also the transport of the serotonin, the reception of it, the re-uptake, and of course the interaction and production of all the other neurotransmitters. For you and I, regular people, concentrate on getting your serotonin up naturally with food and probiotics and the system should regulate itself quite happily.

There is even a disease called Serotonin Syndrome where you have too much serotonin. This disease can only be caused by taking antidepressants, for example overdosing or starting at too high a dose, or adding anti-depressants together. The thing is, you can't naturally get too much serotonin. Even though this syndrome is serious, it will self-regulate fairly quickly if left to nature. Most of us, not all, like drinking alcohol. Alcohol gives a temporary boost to serotonin, that's why we love it.

The Hibernation Theory of Depression

A great article on this theory can be found at goodhealth.co.nz.

(Web source: https://www.goodhealth.co.nz/health-articles/article/tired-hungry-and-sad-relax-youre-hibernating)

Depression is your body shutting down non-essential services in order to survive. Happiness is a non-essential service. Essential services are things like smell, taste, breathing... stuff that keeps you alive in the moment.

When you suffer Depression, your body shuts down some of these 'non-essential services' because it only has enough energy for the essential stuff. Your body is saying, "slow down, take a break, regenerate, I'm not getting what I need, so I have to shut some stuff down. This is the best energy-saving technique that I know of, to force you to do what I want."

Another good analogy is to think of a bear hibernating. The bear has to conserve energy and shut down numerous metabolic processes to make it through the winter without drinking and losing muscle mass. Just try waking a bear from its hibernation and you'll see how grumpy he is. Human Depression is similar. Your body thinks it's starving. It shuts down non-essential services and attempts to conserve energy. Many people with Depression don't want to go out into the world, they just want to hide away; it's kind of like hibernation.

This theory is well expressed in a paper titled: *Metabolic Depression in Hibernation and Major Depression: An Explanatory Theory and an Animal Model of Depression.*

(Web source: https://www.ncbi.nlm.nih.gov/pubmed/16061329)

If this was all we had to do, we'd just take a holiday, chill out, sleep in, and in a month, we'd be right. Well it might help and sometimes it does, but sorry, there's more to it than that. If you keep eating the same, drinking the same, and don't heal your gut, there will be no fix. It's not YOU that needs the holiday and relaxation... it's YOUR GUT. Your gut needs to calm down, relax and strengthen.

There's another aspect to this and I've thought about it all my life. It's the weather. If you lived 200 years ago and you were a farmer or similar (almost everyone), then you lived according to the seasons. You ate seasonally; you gorged in the summer and rested in the winter. When it poured with rain, you stayed in unless there was something urgent you had to do. Here in Queensland, it rains heavily, a lot. It's hot and humid most of the time. But we can't always stay home just because it's raining, or hot, or cold. Modern life demands much more of us. What we all tend to do (me included) is to go about our business regardless of the weather. What that tends to do is fire up the brain, all the time. We have a need in modern society to be switched 'on' all the time. What I am suggesting is that your body was not made for this. It was made to have downtime and uptime: periods of plenty and periods of need: periods of activity and periods of rest. I don't necessarily have the answer to this problem/dilemma. What I'm saying is that in your own life, you should think about it. Maybe your answer to getting downtime is simply sleeping in on Sundays. Maybe it's fasting during Lent or Ramadan. Maybe it's getting drunk every Saturday night: Perhaps its meditation. How about trying this…turn off your mobile phone on a Sunday - sorry, too radical?

There's actually a name for this condition I describe above, it's called Sympathetic Dominance (as opposed to Parasympathetic Dominance). Most people will be familiar with the 'fight or flight' response, which is essentially sympathetic dominance. Due to the 'always on' nature of our world, we often enter into a sympathetic dominance pattern all of the time. Take a truck driver for example; he has to be switched 'on' for an entire 12-hour haul, otherwise he'll crash and die. Our great, great, great grandfathers on the other hand, would run from tigers for thirty minutes and upon reaching safety fall straight to sleep…and they didn't have to do this every day either, just every month or two.

The point I'm trying to make is that the human body and brain is not designed to be 'on' all the time. Our 'normal' state of affairs should be the parasympathetic (resting) state.

If you find yourself in that 'on' position all the time, and it leads to Depression and anxiety, then you should listen to your body and take steps to find some more downtime in your life.

The Inflammation Theory of Depression

Your body is a mixture of inflammation and anti-inflammation. Both are important. Sounds stupid right, but it's not. You NEED inflammation to get rid of old cells…to renew and grow. You also need anti-inflammation to calm and relax … to stabilise. The problem with today's diet and lifestyle is over-emphasis on inflammation. That's why we run around stuffing all these anti-inflammatories into our systems. Take Paracetamol and Ibuprofen for example. The modern diet is so full of inflammatory foods like sugar, omega 6 oils and other stimulants, that there is hardly room for the other stuff. It's like too much excitement, not enough chill…even in our waking lives: too much uptime, not enough downtime. I mean the mobile phone is a great thing, we all love them, but if you had to think about it, would you describe it as inflammatory or anti-inflammatory? I'm not suggesting that you have to meditate, or pray, or find yourself…but I do think you need plenty of downtime if you've had uptime for the last 8 hours straight. If that includes drugs and alcohol, so be it. Take a walk in the forest or just sit and relax on the veranda. You can see the difference between inflammatory and anti-inflammatory now. Inflammation is a CAUSE of Depression; anti-inflammation is a REMEDY for Depression.

Both inflammation and anti-inflammation have their place in society and your body. The problem in the world today, is balancing it all out.

I'm not sure I know the answer to this inflammatory issue, but I will give you a clue... sugar, wheat (gluten), and omega 6 oils, are inflammatory.

Omega 3 oils, aspirin, ibuprofen, fish, and probably meat and butter, are anti-inflammatory. If you look up 'inflammatory' and 'anti-inflammatory' on the internet, I assume you'll get some good advice.

Where our bodies are concerned, inflammation is around us all the time, and we need to balance that with some anti-inflammation. In particular today, our diets are just loaded with inflammatory foods. We need to balance that out.

Here are some foods considered 'Inflammatory':
- Processed snack foods
- Refined grains (flour)
- Processed meats
- Oils from seeds or grains
- Soft drinks, (high sugar content)

Anti-inflammatory foods include:
- Cod liver oil
- Olive oil
- Nuts (peanuts are not real nuts)
- Cheese (unprocessed)
- Red wine
- Dark chocolate

Below is something that I absolutely shouldn't do; quote myself. I'm going to do it anyway because I can…and I love breaking rules. Here's a quote from my own website, it sort of sums up what I want to say about Inflammatory Theory of Depression.

"Inflammation:

Hey almost everyone over the age of forty has got some health problem to deal with today. Some have diabetes, some have obesity, some have thyroid problems, some have wheat allergies, some have nut allergies, some get heartburn, skin conditions, constipation, chronic fatigue syndrome, gout, diverticulitis, Alzheimer's, insomnia. You lucky black dog, you got Depression. Maybe you've got Depression and one of the other problems as well.

What if I told you they are all the same disease - inflammation? I reckon that would shit you off. Well they are. So are the cures.

In one way you're lucky because with diabetes or Alzheimer's for example, when it goes too far it may be untreatable and only manageable.

Depression it is treatable. It can be cured.

A rule of thumb (this not a law)...if you won't put it in your mouth, don't put it on your skin. Well at least think about it first.

Anyway, this is only supposed to be the theories of Depression, not the cures.

Be kind to yourself and balance inflammatory things with anti-inflammatory things."

(Source: Ross Wilkinson)

The Survival Theory of Depression

This is very similar to the Hibernation Theory, but I'm telling you that your body is not just hibernating; it's trying to help you survive.

Homeostasis

Big word, I know, but this word is your best friend. Basically, homeostasis says that your body, the ultimate survival machine, will always look after you and look out for your interests until the day you die. Your body automatically looks out for you in every situation. It just tries to balance everything, the way it likes it, regardless of which way you might push it. It doesn't always win, but it always tries.

So, if you suffer from high blood pressure for example, your body wants high blood pressure for a reason - it's not trying to hurt you and you should let it help you. If your pulse is racing, it's because your body thinks it needs to be racing to defend you from something. I'm not saying that your body never gets it wrong, but your body will always try to protect you from any threat or any perceived threat, and you should let your body do what it does best, PROTECT YOU.

Even when you're hit with Depression, your body is attempting to protect you from something. It might be the food you are eating; it might be the medication you're taking, I don't know your answer. All I know is that your body has your best interests in mind - always.

When you experience a high temperature because you have a fever/infection, this is the body's response to that invader. Your body is hoping that by turning the temperature up, it might kill off the invader. Fevers are generally self- limiting. It's a rare thing that your body, left unchecked, will raise its temperature to dangerous levels. Your body just always tries to protect you. Your body loves you. You are the only one it has to serve. Trust your body.

In The Survival Theory of Depression, I'm saying that your body thinks there is something wrong and it's trying to help you survive. For example, some people with Depression become reluctant to leave the house; they feel tired and lethargic. That's because their body is trying to tell them it needs to stay home and heal. Your body needs to conserve energy. We're all running survival experiments, all of the time. When you have Depression your survival experiment is not working out for you. You have to change the experiment. This doesn't always have to be a massive upheaval. Sometimes it's just a tweak. In the following Chapters you'll find some of the tweaks that helped me, and I sure hope they help you too.

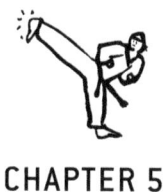

CHAPTER 5

Bacteria and Antibiotics

Some months ago, I met a guy, a TV personality; Current affairs/political commentator. I wanted to 'pitch my idea' to him about fixing Depression. This book was not envisaged at the time. The subject of Depression was in the news quite a bit, and I thought I'd throw my hat in the ring. My personal belief is that most people are on the wrong track with curing Depression. An awful lot of money is spent trying to fix Depression, with very mixed results. In fact, the resources keep expanding, and so does the problem.

I thought, "right…this guy is on TV, he has taken time out to meet me, he probably has a highly-tuned 'Bullshit Radar', and probably gets loads of people pitching him ideas. I'll have to distil my argument down to a few simple things that he can get his head around. And I have to be, or at least appear to be, authentic and sincere. He's more than likely not a scientist or a chemist, just a regular guy trying to make sense of it all like the rest of us." So, I drilled down and found the 'pitch'. I want to share it with you because it's important.

After the usual niceties of sizing each other up, we got down to business. This guy likes philosophy, so I knew that would be important.

My opening line was Newton's Third Law…(you know, Sir Isaac Newton, the guy who invented gravity, the theory of colour, calculus, and momentum, amongst other things) ... *"For every action there is an equal and opposite re-action."* Or as my mate, a millionaire panel beater and philosopher says; *"you never get something for nothing."*

So, in relation to Depression, let's say all medicines have side effects. I hope you will understand this.

My pitch was then, and is now: **"Antibiotics are the primary driver of Depression"**. I decided to put this in big, bold letters because I guess it's the main theme of this book.

Obviously, it's not generally one course of antibiotics that causes Depression, although it can be. And obviously, not everyone gets Depression from Antibiotics.

Usually, it's multiple doses of antibiotics; then there's your diet and lifestyle to take into account, and if you don't replace those all-important good bacteria that live in your gut, then Depression can, and does, occur a lot.

Then I wheeled out the following: *Antibiotic Exposure and the Risk for Depression, Anxiety, or Psychosis: A Nested Case-control Study.* It presented a million English people, showing their likelihood of suffering Depression was 25% higher if they took one course of antibiotics in the past 10 years. Two to five courses then increased their likelihood of suffering Depression to 50% higher again.
(Web source: https://www.ncbi.nlm.nih.gov/pubmed/26580313)

Now most people don't really get how scientific papers work, I have plenty of trouble with them myself, but when you see stats like that, you really should pay attention.

Just to explain those stats in 'regular people' talk, imagine that there were three groups with 300,000 people in each group. The first group didn't take any antibiotics in 10 years; 30,000 of them ended up with Depression (10%).

In the second group of 300,000, those who took only one course of antibiotics, there would be 37,500 cases of Depression (25% more, or 12.5% of 300,000). The third group took between two to five courses of antibiotics; 45,000 cases of Depression (50% more, or 15% of 300,000). Often you'll see scientific studies where there is a 10% shift one way or the other, and it possibly means nothing. A 50% shift is massive and needs attention. It isn't proof of any concept, but I believe you should pay attention anyway. This is not the only study coming to the same conclusion.

So, my point is: <u>The 'Primary Driver' of Depression is antibiotics</u>.

Antibiotics are wonderful, life-saving drugs, and you should take them if your doctor says so, but that doesn't mean that there aren't unintended consequences. I mean your doctor is there to relieve your current ailment and keep you alive for the next few weeks. After that, it's your responsibility.

Antibiotics have side effects, even if they take a long time to show up, and the broader the spectrum, the greater the likelihood of unintended consequences. The more of them you take, the more damage you do to your gut. These babies kill off the invading bacteria, but they kill off a lot of stuff that you need as well.

You can't completely reverse the side effects of antibiotics, but you can do an awful lot, easily, to offset them. In this book I hope to show you how.

If your doctor says take these antibiotics, then take them, or not, that's up to you. I take antibiotics when I have to. Just be aware that they can help you and harm you, at the same time.

Classic example: Dropping the bomb on Hiroshima was tragic if you happened to live in Hiroshima. But it quite possibly helped the rest of us and shortened the war by many months, even years. Hiroshima may have had some bad people in it, but there were an awful lot of good ones too. Antibiotics are like an atom bomb in your gut. They kill stuff, bad stuff, but they kill good stuff too. There's a lot of collateral damage.

The good bacteria that live in your gut make serotonin for you. Serotonin is a chemical in your body that makes you feel good. If you seriously interfere with your serotonin production, you get Depression. There are many other ways to interfere with Serotonin production, other than antibiotics. We'll discuss that shortly, but <u>antibiotics are my number one</u>.

An easy way to counter the adverse effects of antibiotics is probiotics. Probiotics come in medicinal form, like pills and powders, but there are also 'natural' probiotics like fermented foods, including sauerkraut, yoghurt, beer, wine, Kombucha, buttermilk, Kimchi, Kefir, raw cheese, and foods that have prebiotic fibre. Prebiotic fibre feeds the good bacteria, like properly cooked potatoes, vegetables, long-fermented nutritious breads, beans, and fruit. Look after your good bacteria and Depression will reduce or disappear.

Just to show that I'm bipartisan about this, there are many other things that contribute to Depression, but most of them are 'bacteria killing' things. Chlorine kills bacteria. Detergent kills bacteria. Hot water kills bacteria. Sunscreens kill bacteria. Refrigerators kill bacteria. Soap kills bacteria. The cleanliness of modern life kills bacteria. Bacteria are not all bad. I'd like to say that many bacteria you will encounter in life are good guys. Many of them are trying to help you.

Stop killing your good bacteria and they will help you.

Okay, I suspect I'm losing you here, or your eyes are glazing over. Let's take a quick trip to the 'Land of Bacteria'.

Bacteria

Most people, I would suggest, think of bacteria (germs if you like) as being inherently bad. Bacterial infections cause illness, for example food poisoning, cholera, pneumonia, bubonic plague, tuberculosis. We try to keep our houses clean by using chemicals and water to 'kill germs.' We wipe down surfaces with chemicals that 'kill 99.99% of all germs.' We add chlorine to our water with the prime intention to kill germs (bacteria).

Florence Nightingale brought tremendous change to hospitals and survival rates when she began making cleanliness the norm, rather than the exception. She was a bacteria killer.

No doubt our understanding of bacteria has increased exponentially in the last 100 years, in fact bacteria were only 'discovered' in 1670. It then took hundreds of years to find out what bacteria actually 'did.'

Once we found out what bacteria 'did' in about 1860, we then set about trying to kill them all off; e.g. pasteurisation, chlorination, fluoridation, antibiotics, antibacterials. We have been on a mission since Pasteur (1822 to 1895) to kill and eliminate bacteria with industrial chemicals, processes and medicines. We have gone to war with bacteria. There is actually a name for this war, it's called 'The Germ Theory of Disease'. The Germ Theory of Disease is largely correct, but there is a problem. Many of the 'germs' are double agents, and many of them are permanently on our side.

We have won many important battles against bacteria, and we've slowly entered an arms race with them, but we can never win. I mean you would have heard of Antibiotic resistance. We wheeled out penicillin, probably the greatest medical invention, so far, (first used about 1945) and bacteria have been biding their time and slowly building up their arsenals. Antibiotics are like the nuclear weapon against bacteria. Nuclear weapons are either the greatest force of destruction ever seen, or the greatest source of peace ever seen in the world, depending on your perspective. Possibly a bit of both. We are finally learning that bacteria are at one time, a great scourge, but greatly beneficial as well. Unfortunately, we have only learned about the therapeutic value of bacteria recently, and we now know that bacteria are formidable enemies, and our friends at the same time. Some bacteria just want to help us. This book is largely about re-establishing our friendships with good bacteria and taking back our health by allowing those good bacteria to help us.

So what do bacteria do? The answer is <u>everything</u>. Once the planet was formed about 5 billion years ago, it probably took a billion years or so before bacteria 'spontaneously' turned up. Bacteria then evolved into all sorts of life forms and even created the atmosphere. But let's say that you believe in creationism, where God created everything. That works too. God created the planet first, then the bacteria to make the atmosphere, then animals, plants and then human life. That makes just as much sense, and I mean that sincerely, even though I believe in the traditional version of evolution. Even if you believe in the literal interpretation of the bible; that God created the world in seven days, then bacteria would have been on Day 2. Humans turned up on Day 6 then God rested on Day 7.

The point is here, bacteria are important to all life, the planet and certainly pretty important to human life. If you killed all the bacteria in and on your body right now, I suspect your lifespan would be measured in hours, not days.

Most animals that we are familiar with breathe in oxygen and breathe out carbon dioxide. Plants do the opposite; they breathe in carbon dioxide and breathe out oxygen. Bacteria are not restricted to that at all. Bacteria are like the LGBTIQ+ community, very diverse.

Girls like boys, boys like boys, girls like girls, girls dress as boys, and vice versa. Some bacteria can even reproduce asexually (without a partner). These guys are really versatile.

Some bacteria like oxygen (aerobes) and some don't like oxygen (anaerobes). Some will tolerate oxygen but prefer not to (facultative anaerobes). Others will tolerate carbon dioxide but prefer not to (facultative aerobes), and some live in places we thought were completely uninhabitable, like your petrol tank, or near volcanic vents in the seabed. Some bacteria thrive in strong acid and drink it like Kool Aid. Bacteria are extremely adaptable and constantly change to suit their environment.

Bacteria and Humans

Bacteria and humans live together like the lyrics of Stevie Wonder and Paul McCartney's song; *"Ebony, Ivory, living in perfect harmony."* Well usually it is, but not always. Reality sometimes gets in the way of a good song lyric. Humans, bacteria, fungi, parasites, and viruses live in a peaceful yet savage co-existence with each other, like a rainforest or a coral reef. So long as you don't interfere too much, the whole system works perfectly happily. Every now and then an invader who doesn't know the rules gets involved. In this instance, a defence must be mounted.

The 'Not So Mythical' Land of Bacteria

Bacteria are like tiny little animals. I mean a million of them would fit on the head of a pin, that kind of tiny. Bacteria are single celled animals. They are usually not classed as animals but as organisms. Bacteria are everywhere. They're in the air, water, the soil, on your skin, in your hair, your stomach, your food, and in your intestines. There are bucket loads of bacteria in and on you right now. How's this? There are more bacterial cells on your hands right now than there are people on the planet! A healthy person is home to approximately 50-100 trillion bacterial cells. Most of these bacteria are contained in your colon. The colon is the last two metres of pipe before your arse (ass for Americans). Most of the dry weight of your stool (your poo) is dead bacteria. Some bacteria in your stool are alive too. When you interfere with these bacteria, as we are all good at doing, then your chances of suffering Depression increase. Bacteria, the ones inside you and on you, are mostly good and helpful. There are always a few unhelpful ones. It's just like people. Most people are good and helpful, some just hang around and don't seem to do much, and others are downright unhelpful. The trick, just like life itself, is to hang out with the helpful ones as much as possible, and limit the unhelpful ones. Most of the bacteria you have right now in and on you are good bacteria and are trying to help you.

Examples of helpful bacteria include E. coli, Lactobacillus, and Bifidobacteria. In fact a healthy person is home to 1000 species of bacteria.

Every now and then bad bacteria turn up, and you need to defeat them. Here's an example: food poisoning, which is often caused by salmonella bacteria. Salmonella makes you really sick. Then your body fights back, doing everything it can to expel this poison. Vomiting, shitting, raising your temperature, whatever your body can do to get rid of this toxin. Usually, your body wins…yay! Then all returns to normal. 'Normal' in this case is normal levels of good bacteria.

Antibiotics are medicines that kill bacteria. Literally translated, 'antibiotic' means 'against life.' So, antibiotics kill bacteria. Again, yay! It's a great thing…saves our lives occasionally.

Hey, my doctor once said:

> *"If you get the flu or a cold (quite different things) then I could give you antibiotics and you will probably recover in two weeks. On the other hand, if I give you nothing, it could take as long as fourteen days!"*

That's obviously a joke, but really, antibiotics are fantastic. The problem is that they do have side effects, and one of those side effects is Depression. It just might not show up for weeks, or even years after you take them.

I'm attempting to give a broad brush here, because the technical details are ahead in the upcoming chapters. Let me give you some food for thought on the dangers of antibiotics.

Just before I launch into some specific cases, read this.

Drug and Antibiotic Information and Side Effects

The side effects of the drugs that you are taking are listed on the leaflet included. But who reads them? Just a heads-up, drug information leaflets are often not included with medicines in Australia anymore. The reasons are fair enough. Firstly, as I mentioned, no one reads them anyway. Secondly, your pharmacist can supply that information, but you have to care enough to ask. Thirdly, all of this information is available online now. Have a look on the box of the next prescription drug you purchase, especially antibiotics. The drug companies don't even provide their website addresses. They really don't want you looking into the side effects of their drugs. They'd prefer that you simply take it and shut up. I mean everyone sticks their website address on their packaging these days, but not drug companies, isn't that strange? I'd strongly encourage you, before taking any drug, to familiarise yourself with what the drug actually does, and what its side effects are. Also be aware that the side effects are not always listed in order of how often they occur.

Specific Antibiotics/Quinolones

There's at least one class of antibiotics that I vow never to take again, unless I'm on my deathbed with infection. They're called Quinolones. If you are prescribed these, I recommend you do your research first. Some Quinolones carry a 'Black Box Warning' in the USA, which includes mental health side effects that may, or may not be permanent. A Black Box warning is the highest warning possible. It can mean that the side effects may include risks of psychiatric episodes and suicidal ideation.

I took Quinolones twenty years ago and I had issues. I called it a 'nervous breakdown.' My mother also took them in the last few years of her life, and she experienced hallucinations.

The ADF (Australian Defence Force) recently conducted 'Information nights' for military personnel who had concerns about the side effects of Quinolones. Numerous soldiers took them while serving in Malaria-prone countries. I don't know what the outcome of those information nights was.

This is a quote from The Australian Department of Defence website:

> *"What are the side effects of Mefloquine?*
>
> *For most people taking mefloquine side effects are minor and the medication is generally well tolerated. When taken for malaria prevention, the predominant side effects are neuropsychiatric – sleep problems, vivid dreams, anxiety, and depressive symptoms. Trouble sleeping and vivid dreams are the most common of these, occurring in around 13% of people.*
>
> *Uncommonly, people taking mefloquine can experience agitation, restlessness, mood swings, panic attacks, confusion, hallucinations, aggression, psychosis and suicidal ideation. These symptoms occur in less than 1% of people taking mefloquine.*
>
> *Other neurological symptoms, such as dizziness and headache are relatively common, occurring in up to 10% of people. Uncommonly (less than 1%), balance problems and seizures can occur. People who have, or have had, any mental health condition or seizure disorder should not take mefloquine."*

NOTE: At the time of printing, this reference has now been removed from the ADF website. It's possible to access the TGA (Therapeutic Goods Administration) in Australia to read the side effects of Mefloquine/Lariam. I don't have permission to reprint them here, but I can assure you that it isn't written in plain English...hardly what I'd describe as 'consumer friendly' either.

So if you want to know the side effects for Mefloquine, you'll have to look it up yourself.

Just another comment from me...not all adverse effects are reported!

I know when I had my problem with Fluoroquinolones, I had no idea that an antibiotic prescribed by a doctor could possibly have these side effects. When I reported my mother's hallucinations to her doctors, they refused to believe that an antibiotic could cause these problems, even though hallucinations are listed as a side effect in the official literature. When you see that adverse reactions are reported in 13% of cases, my bet is the actual number is much higher, maybe 50%. I mean if you are a soldier facing an enemy, and carrying an automatic weapon, and you experience terrible dreams, are you going to report that to your Drill Sergeant? Unlikely. Don't be fooled by medical statistics, they're only a guide...at best.

I was just about to complete this book when COVID-19 took the world by storm. One of the proposed cures is Hyroxychloroquine (HyC). HyC is not chloroquine or Mefloquine. I've been told that HyC is less harsh than chloroquine, but it is a fluoroquinolone. Again, if I was on my death-bed I'd take it, otherwise I wouldn't. Apparently it's only really dangerous when taken for long periods, like if you're working or serving in a malaria-prone area. Even then, I believe it's being phased out. The official reason: its no longer effective for chronic malaria. My theory is that the side effects are just too common, too severe, and often enough, irreversible.

Cephalexin

Cephalexin is sold under the original name of Keflex, and also under generic names. I'll devote some more time to the issue of generics later, but be careful of generics.

My mother had a dose of cephalexin shortly before she died. She did not die from cephalexin, nor any complications from it.

She called me at 6am one morning. I could tell from the phone call that she was hallucinating. She described people running around outside the house, trying to get in, and she wanted me to call the police. I was obviously concerned and asked my wife to accompany me to my mother's house, because I had no idea what would happen when I arrived. 30 minutes later we were in her house and all was calm, as I suspected. She, my mother, had a perfectly normal and civil conversation with my wife and I, but she was still hallucinating at the same time. She asked why these people were trying to hurt her, but there was no one else there. She also asked what the woman at the end of the bed wanted. Again, no one there. All the while she was having a conversation with my wife about the royal family, and talking to me about Australia's most successful racehorse, 'Winx'. She knew more about the horse than I did. My mother had all of her marbles, even in her 90's, but she was hallucinating throughout our entire conversation.

Mum also experienced quite a bit of pain, which I'd describe as nerve pain. That's described in the side effects literature too. She went off in an ambulance to the hospital and stayed for a week.

Whilst she was there, I had a look through her medications and discovered the Cephalexin, (generic) and began looking into the side effects. Here's some official literature I found, after some research.

"Cephalexin side effects:

Seek emergency medical help if you have signs of an allergic reaction to Cephalexin: hives; difficulty breathing; swelling of your face, lips, tongue, or throat.

Call your doctor at once if you have:

- *Severe stomach pain, diarrhoea that is watery or bloody;*
- *Jaundice (yellowing of the skin or eyes);*
- *Easy bruising, unusual bleeding (nose, mouth, vagina, or rectum), purple or red pinpoint spots under your skin;*
- *Little or no urination;*

- *Agitation, confusion, hallucinations; or*
- *Severe skin reaction-fever, sore throat, swelling in your face or tongue, burning in your eyes, skin pain followed by a red or purple skin rash that spreads (especially in the face or upper body) and causes blistering and peeling.*

(Web source: https://www.drugs.com/cephalexin.html)

There had been a previous incident concerning my mother in 2018. She was in hospital at the time, injured from falling into the river. She contracted a rare bacteria that flourishes after rain. Normally it infects fish, and only occasionally, humans. While trying to find the offending bacteria, numerous antibiotics were administered, but they didn't stop the infection. One day I was visiting her when she reported that there had been a man outside her room in the hospital, during the night, and she was quite scared. Her room was on the fourth floor of a new hospital, with sheer glass walls. The guy must have been very determined to peep on my 90-year-old mother to scale the glass walls at night. Maybe he was just a very dedicated window cleaner…who knows.

It's possible that the hallucination thing is more prevalent in older people, whose guts are already compromised. I have certainly had that reported to me by others on the same drug, with similar experiences. What I'm trying to say is that there are psychological, as well as physical consequences of taking antibiotics. Whatever affects the gut, affects the mind.

Here's a quote from *Medical Diagnosis* magazine:

> *"Antibiotics are essential for curing an array of conditions, but they may also be responsible for disrupting cognitive function in patients.*
>
> *Although mental confusion can be caused by some medications, such as opiates and sleeping pills, most people wouldn't suspect that antibiotics would make the list. However, researchers from Brigham and Women's Hospital (BWH) in Boston found that antibiotic use can lead to delirium, accompanied by hallucinations and agitation.*

The study included 391 patients over seven decades who had developed delirium and other brain problems after being treated with antibiotics.

Fifty-four different antibiotics from 12 different classes were reported, including sulfonamides and ciprofloxacin, as well as intravenous varieties like penicillin and cefepime. As described in the journal **Neurology**, of the 391 patients:

- 47% had delusions or hallucinations
- 15% had involuntary muscle twitching
- 14% had seizures
- 5% had loss control of body movements

In addition, EEG (electroencephalogram) tests revealed that 70% of patients had abnormal electrical activity in the brain.

People who have delirium are more likely to have other complications, go into a nursing home instead of going home after being in the hospital and are more likely to die than people who do not develop delirium."

(Web source: https://www.mdmag.com/medical-news/penicillin-other-common-antibiotics-can-cause-delirium)

And this article below from the *International Journal of Clinical Pharmacology and Therapeutics*, published in 2002.

"Hallucinations with therapeutic doses of clarithromycin:

OBJECTIVE:
Hallucinations caused by adverse reactions to medication are not uncommon and a wide variety of drugs may be involved. We present a case of hallucinations caused by therapeutic doses of oral clarithromycin (500mg b.i.d).

CASE REPORT:
A 32-year-old woman attended the Emergency Department of the hospital with severe visual hallucinations together with marked

anxiety and nervousness following the second dose of clarithromycin, which was the only medication she was taking. The antibiotic was identified as the possible cause of the clinical manifestations and was stopped immediately. The patient did not require hospitalization and was discharged a few hours later with no signs of neurological disturbances. Clarithromycin was substituted by amoxycillin-clavulanic acid (500/125 mg) t.i.d.

CONCLUSIONS:
The temporal relationship between commencement of antibiotic therapy and the appearance of hallucinations, together with the fact that the symptoms disappeared once the antibiotic was suspended, support a causal relationship between clarithromycin and the hallucinations. Further support for a causal relationship was obtained by application of Naranjo's algorithm which gave a likelihood level for causality of PROBABLE."

I'm saying that Depression is primarily driven by antibiotics...but I would also assert that usually the antibiotics need assistance to cause Depression. The assistance is other anti-bacterial agents like chlorine in the water supply, fluoride in water and toothpastes, antimicrobial agents like triclosan and triclocarban, and a poor diet, or a diet with preservatives, synthetic sugars and cheap cooking oils. In short, a bacteria-killing diet. It's a matter of whether a person rebuilds their gut bacteria or not, after taking antibiotics, that makes the difference.

The problem of course is that you can't 'un-take' the antibiotics, but what you can do is rebuild the gut and the gut bacteria by improving your diet, and taking supplements that encourage the good bacteria to return. Fortunately, this can be done rather quickly in many cases. In the following chapters I'll aim to tell you how.

Not only Bacteria, but Yeast, Fungi, Viruses, Worms and Parasites

All of these life forms, except for worms and parasites, are found in and on you all of the time. You'd better get used to it. Worms and parasites can be very common also, take India for example, worms and parasites are more common than not…and there are an awful lot of Indians. These life forms are not always hugely detrimental to a person's health, and occasionally there are benefits. Your chances of going through life without worms and parasites, is low. If you lived the rest of your life with worms and parasites, there is little evidence to show that your life would be worse, or shorter. It depends on the type of parasite or worm of course.

Yeast, fungi, and viruses are part of you all the time. Like the bacteria mentioned above, there's much more to learn about these life forms and the science is still in its infancy.

One of the most common types of detrimental yeast/fungi that is found in humans is Candida Albicans. I suggest that we all have it. It's not a great problem, unless it overgrows. Candida overgrows due to antibiotics and a high sugar diet, amongst other things. Its overgrowth causes an increase in detrimental chemicals like uric acid (causes gout) and candida (causes thrush) in women, among other diseases.

I don't have much expertise with Candida, but I suggest that it doesn't only cause physical symptoms, but psychological symptoms as well. I've seen it.

Parasites

By definition, a parasite is something that takes from you, and doesn't contribute anything back. What I would like to say is that your likelihood of acquiring a parasite at some time in your life is extremely high. Often, they go away on their own, but not always. Parasites can also cause psychological and physical ailments. The best way to keep parasites at bay is to maintain a healthy diet and a strong microbiome (lots of good bacteria).

Worms

Worms are such a fun subject that I have read whole books about. The point is, these guys are very common and not always detrimental. In fact, Pinworms are now used to improve symptoms of gluten sensitivity and some other allergies. There are people who suffer allergic conditions that actually intentionally infect themselves with worms, and sometimes get relief from those allergies. NOTE: I'm not suggesting that if you have worms, it contributes to Depression.

Viruses

Just as I was about to print this book, the Coronavirus reared its ugly head. It can make you a little sick, or cause death in some situations. The thing is, not all viruses kill you, and some of them are beneficial. We don't yet know how bad this coronavirus really is. It may turn out to be something that helps us. I doubt it, but that's not the point. Not all viruses are harmful and not all viruses weaken you. It's the same with bacteria.

You are not 'Just For You'

What I'm saying is that your body is not just for you. Your body is a thriving ecosystem for all sorts of other life forms. This is not unique to humans; this is the normal state of affairs. What we need to do is encourage the good, helpful life forms and discourage the not-so-helpful ones. It's easier than you might think, but you first need to accept the fact that there is more to you than meets the eye. If you help the good life forms, like beneficial bacteria, they will help you in return; they want to help. You are their home and what helps you, helps them, mostly. If they wanted you dead or depressed, they could help you do that, but there's no fun in it. The things that live in and on you, are primarily interested in their own survival, and that depends on you staying alive, mostly.

Depression before Antibiotics

I've courageously stated that antibiotics are the primary driver of Depression. Where does that leave me, prior to the invention of antibiotics? I mean Depression existed before antibiotics were even invented.

Winston Churchill famously suffered from Depression and that was well before antibiotics. There are plenty of natural antibiotics. Garlic has antimicrobial properties, so does honey, black walnut, ginger and oregano, liquorice, and arsenic. There are dozens of them. I mean I don't know what caused Winston's problem. We will never know. Maybe it was a parasite.

Antibiotics are ubiquitous today and they are much stronger and more devastating to your gut bacteria than natural bacterial-killing substances. One of the primary purposes of the very strong hydrochloric acid in your stomach is to kill bacteria before it has a chance to get further down into your system. Hydrochloric acid is a backup system, a protection racket in your body. It's there to protect you from the high chance that a bad bacteria or virus makes its way into your digestive system. So, before antibiotics, there were plenty of antimicrobial agents around that would help kill off gut bacteria. There were also lots of bad, harmful bacteria that occasionally made their way past the stomach and into your digestive system; cholera for example.

You'll read later that people who drank Gin (you know 'crying in your Gin') often drank Gin with tonic water. Tonic water is made with Quinine (the tonic). Quinine is a medicine that wards off Malaria. Quinine is a well-known depression-causing compound. In this chapter I also write about Quinolone antibiotics and how they cause neuropsychological effects. The 'Quin' in Quinolone is quinine, a wholly natural extract from tree bark. Quinine has been used for hundreds of years. If you suffer from Depression, and happen to be a G&T drinker, then just drink Gin and lemonade for a week and see if that helps, it might.

Anyway, the story is, that before antibiotics, there were plenty of natural antibiotics and medicines and bad bacteria that may have been applied and ingested either accidentally or purposely. Sometimes these may have caused Depression.

A new 'superfood' is Quinoa (unrelated to Quinine). It's very high in natural saponins. Saponins are soap-like substances found in plants. Indigenous tribes used plants containing Saponins to catch fish. Aborigines would dam a section of river and then scatter plants on the water containing saponins. The saponins stun or kill the fish, in other words poison the fish. What actually happens is that the bubbles produced by the soap, stops the fish from breathing. Then the aborigines found it easy to harvest the fish. We now willingly eat these natural poisons. I'm not saying don't eat Quinoa, I'm saying that you should try to eliminate or reduce the natural poisons in these foods, otherwise they can affect your gut bacteria and therefore your mental health. By the way, with Quinoa, what you do is pressure cook it, or ferment it, and then boil the crap out of it before you eat it. That kills off the saponins, but retains most of the other 'good' natural proteins.

So, Depression existed in historical times before antibiotics. I suggest that the mechanisms were possibly the same. Gut bacteria died because of invading bacteria or natural antibiotics. Gut bacteria were not replaced by food or other means, and serotonin-producing bacteria were reduced. My further assertion is that Depression occurred historically, just a lot less...a LOT less!

Bacteria control your Behaviour

Bacteria and other micro life forms in and around your body have far more control over you than you would like to think. I don't want to scare you or make you think that you are not a unique individual, but in the end, these micro bastards have more influence over you than you care to contemplate. This will be the most controversial subject that I raise in the book. I'm still grappling with it myself. You are not in control of things nearly as much as you think you are. These micro guys have lots to say.

Let me tell you a quick story about Toxoplasma Gondii, a common parasite (i.e. not a bacteria, but a protozoa).

Unless you're a cat, you don't have to worry about this too much. It's just an example.

Toxoplasma Gondii is a parasite that lives and breeds in cats. Toxo will live in almost any mammal, but it can only reproduce in cats. Don't ask me why, I'm just a dumb engineer.

Toxo G can run around all over the world, but until it gets into a cat, it can't reproduce sexually. It hangs around in mammals, like mice, but it cannot reproduce in mice, only pass from mouse to mouse. That's no fun.

Once Toxoplasma gets into a mouse, it needs to get into a cat. The best way for Toxo to get into a cat is to have the mouse eaten by a cat. The best way for a mouse to be eaten by a cat is for the mouse to hang around cats; not something a mouse does willingly. Once Toxo gets hold of a mouse, it needs to make the mouse 'cat friendly', and it does. I don't know the exact mechanism here, but I suspect it's something to do with the neurotransmitter GABA, and perhaps Dopamine. Instead of the mice scurrying from place to place, the Toxo-infected mouse becomes much more outgoing and friendly, chilled out. Chances of the mouse being eaten by a cat increase exponentially. Apparently, the mice actually start hanging around the cats' food bowls, and are attracted by the cats' scent. The mouse has become a risk taker.

Now, I know you're thinking, "It's just a stupid mouse, that doesn't happen with humans." Well funnily enough, it does. There was a study undertaken on Toxoplasma Gondii in humans. Not really humans, but university students, close enough. What they found was the students who were infected with Toxoplasma Gondii, were much more likely to pursue careers where 'risk taking' was involved, for example more likely to study business, than science or engineering.

Here are excerpts from two articles on *biomedcentral.com*:

> *"Mind altering microbes: Can Toxoplasma gondii infection increase entrepreneurship?*
>
> *Toxoplasma gondii infection is thought to alter the personalities of infected individuals (whether rats or humans) by increasing risk-taking behaviors. Studies have shown that this can lead to more accidents, but on the flip side Stefanie Johnson and colleagues recently showed that this risk taking tendency can lead to increased entrepreneurial behaviors. However, before we start infecting ourselves with the parasite, be warned that increased entrepreneurial-type behavior does not necessarily result in successful businesses or wealth."*

And this one...

> *"Effects of Toxoplasma on Human Behavior:*
>
> *The personality of infected men showed lower superego strength (rule consciousness) and higher vigilance (factors G and L on Cattell's 16PF). Thus, the men were more likely to disregard rules and were more expedient, suspicious, jealous, and dogmatic. The personality of infected women, by contrast, showed higher warmth and higher superego strength (factors A and G on Cattell's 16PF), suggesting that they were more warm hearted, outgoing, conscientious, persistent, and moralistic. Both men and women had significantly*

higher apprehension (factor O) compared with the uninfected controls."

Here's another from the *US National Library of Medicine*:

"Can the common brain parasite, Toxoplasma gondii, influence human culture?

Toxoplasma gondii is a single-celled brain parasite spread by cats. Our feline companions are its preferred home and only in their bodies can it mature and reproduce. So like most parasites, T.gondii has a complex life cycle designed to get it into its final host. If it finds itself in another animal, it travels to the brain and changes the host's behaviour to maximise its chances of ending up in a cat. For rodents, this means being eaten and infected individuals are less fearful of cats and more active, making them easier prey.

Carriers tend to show long-term personality changes that are small but statistically significant. Women tend to be more intelligent, affectionate, social and more likely to stick to rules. Men on the other hand tend to be less intelligent, but are more loyal, frugal and mild-tempered. The one trait that carriers of both genders share is a higher level of neuroticism – they are more prone to guilt, self-doubt and insecurity.

In individual cases, these effects may seem quirky or even charming but across populations, they can have a global power. T.gondii infection is extremely common and rates vary greatly from country to country. While only 7% of Brits carry the parasite, a much larger 67% of Brazilians are infected. Given that the parasite alters behaviour, infection on this scale could lead to sizeable differences in the general personalities of people of different nationalities. This is exactly what Lafferty found."

Gut and Personality Study:

"Study of human personality vs gut diversity and abundance:

KEY FINDINGS:
Gut diversity and also abundance or lack of particular species are predictive of certain behavioural characteristics, for instance reaction to stress, anxiety, depression, sociability, degree of extroversion.

Antibiotic treatment in the last 6 months had a major influence on gut diversity.

Probiotic and prebiotic foods had a much stronger influence on gut diversity than probiotic and prebiotic supplements.

Gut diversity had a strong correlation with overall general health.

Fish consumption was related to diversity of gut microbiome."

In conclusion, the article states:

"Finally, it is pertinent to reflect on the ways in which our modern-day living may provide a perfect storm for dysbiosis of the gut. We lead stressful lives with fewer social interactions and less time spent with nature, our diets are typically deficient in fibre, we inhabit oversanitized environments and are dependent on antibiotic treatments. All these factors can influence the gut microbiome and so may be affecting our behaviour and psychological wellbeing in currently unknown ways."

(Web source: www.sciencedirect.com/science/article/pii/S2452231719300181? via%3Dihub)

Bifidobacteria make you Calm

We're getting a bit too nitty gritty here, but bacteria can and do influence your behaviour. I don't know to what extent that occurs, but I suggest that the mechanism is through the production of neurotransmitters.

I further suggest by way of example that people with higher levels of Bifidobacteria will tend to be calmer and more relaxed due to higher levels of GABA, the calming neurotransmitter. I've seen this with my own children, when I give them bifido probiotics; they are more relaxed and happier. I've seen it in adults too. Even a friend of mine, after taking probiotics for a week, his family commented on how much more fun he was to be around. The changes are often subtle, but they are there.

Some years ago, I asked my naturopath if it were normal for Depression to 'turn around' so quickly, after taking probiotics (which is what happened to me). She said it would 'normally' take a month or so. Then she informed me that in the case of children, sometimes it only takes hours. Again, I've seen this myself. I gave a 4-year-old some weak, kiddy probiotics. I saw her personality change within 30 minutes. She wasn't depressed initially, but she was awfully shy and wouldn't speak to anyone outside her own family. Within a few days that all changed. Everyone noticed and commented on it, though they didn't know she was taking probiotics. Now that she's on regular probiotics, she's a chatterbox and you can't shut her up. Her anxiety has disappeared.

At the risk of being boring, I've also seen it with a dog. After one dose of probiotics, the dog was calmer and nicer to be around. It was a large dog and it took about half a day to kick in.

Candida

Candida is a kind of yeast. Yeast and bacteria are different, but to us non-microbiologists, it probably doesn't matter much. Yeasts are tiny little plants. Candida Albicans is extremely common in humans and I'd suggest that perhaps all of us have it. It's not a great problem, until it 'overgrows'. That's common enough too... and it causes thrush, amongst other problems. That's the problem with Candida, it just shows up in so many places and has wildly varying symptoms. Antibiotics and high sugar diets may well be the cause. Antibiotics kill the bacteria that compete with Candida and sugar feeds it. Candida loves sugar.

Candida lets you know when it's hungry, because you get hungry... hungry for sugar. The Candida is influencing your behaviour. You feed the Candida sugar, it grows more, and you need more sugar. I'm not saying all sugar eating is to feed Candida, just that it can, and does, influence your behaviour. Candida overgrowth can also be associated with Depression and anxiety. If you have visible signs of Candida, like white spots on the skin, nail fungus, itchy bottom, irritable bowel, and you suffer from Depression or anxiety, I'd encourage you to get tested for Candida. It's another gut issue that may lead to Depression. Who would have thought?

Fibre

It isn't talked about as much as it used to be, but fibre is really important to feed your bacteria. We'll discuss this later on, in detail. The bacteria in your colon eat fibre. It's often said that a high fibre diet makes you feel fuller for longer. You don't need to eat as much. When your bacteria get fed, they're happy. When they're underfed, they are not. When you eat a low fibre diet, which is common, your bacteria aren't being fed, so they send messages to eat more. If you then eat another low fibre meal or snack, they still don't get fed, so they keep sending you messages that you're hungry. Just try it once or twice and see what happens. Add 5 or 10 grams of fibre, like apple pectin, slippery elm, gelatin, unmodified potato starch, or baked beans, and see what happens.

The simple message here is that bacteria influence your behaviour. Keep them happy and you will be happier.

Get Down and Dirty

Natural soil is loaded with bacteria. Bacteria break down vegetation and turn it into nitrogen to feed other plants. If you dig in the dirt, the bacteria get into your skin. Generally, this is a good thing, but who regularly digs in the dirt today? Almost none of us I'm guessing.

About twenty years ago, I did quite a bit of landscaping. I met a number of people working in nurseries, dealing with plants. I noticed how they all seemed to be calm and happy. What I mean is that I noticed 'as a group' they were far more calm in comparison to other people I dealt with in business. I put it down to the fact that they were working with living things, and watching stuff grow is fulfilling. That was a decent theory. I now know it wasn't that simple. It's the bacteria in the soil that makes them happy. Bacteria are absorbed into their system, causing serotonin and GABA formation. Here are a few anecdotes about soil and bacteria, and a dilemma to solve.

Mycobacterium Vaccae

Certain strains of Mycobacteria cause tuberculosis, a nasty disease. Mycobacterium Vaccae doesn't cause tuberculosis. M.Vaccae is found in the soil. A brilliant English scientist was working in Africa with M.Vaccae and found that it cured his Depression. Most of his family also suffered from Depression. He gave the M.Vaccae to those particular family members and their Depression left. Apparently, whatever he did was against the law for some reason, I think he wasn't supposed to import the bacteria into England, and wasn't supposed to infect other humans with it, so it didn't extend beyond his own family.

M.Vaccae is now undergoing trials for curing Depression.

This is a quote from *Wikipedia*:

> *"Research areas being pursued with regard to killed Mycobacterium vaccae vaccine include immunotherapy for allergic asthma, cancer, depression, leprosy, psoriasis, dermatitis, eczema and tuberculosis.*
>
> *A research group at Henry Wellcome Laboratories for Integrative Neuroscience and Endocrinology, University of Bristol, Bristol, England, UK has shown that Mycobacterium vaccae stimulated a newly discovered group of neurons, increased levels of serotonin*

*and decreased levels of anxiety in mice. Other researchers fed
live Mycobacterium vaccae to mice, then measured their ability to
navigate a maze compared to control mice not fed the bacteria."*

According to Dorothy Matthews, who conducted the research with
Susan Jenks at the Sage Colleges, Troy, New York, USA:

*"Mice that were fed live M. vaccaenavigated the maze twice as fast
and with less demonstrated anxiety behaviors as control mice.
Mycobacterium vaccae is in the same genus as Mycobacterium
tuberculosis, the bacterium which causes tuberculosis."*

Maybe, don't wait for the trials. That could take years. Just go and get
your hands dirty. Hey...people have been doing it for years, and it
didn't kill them. Just a quick warning: It doesn't work with potting mix.
There can be harmful bacteria in that stuff.

Children playing in Sand

Don't the kids love getting in the sand and the mud? Could it be that
there's something tiny living in the soil that gets into their system and
makes them feel good? In Queensland we have a mud festival once a
year, where everyone gets to play in the stuff. Apparently it's great for
kids' health. Apparently it improves their immune systems and gives
them a cheerier outlook. I wonder why?

The Farmer Dilemma

There's an awful lot of Depression among farmers in today's society.
Farmers get dirty all the time and connect to the soil. This would easily
seem to counter my arguments above about getting your hands dirty. I
wish I knew the answer, but I can only speculate.

Perhaps much of the soil that farmers encounter today is laced with
chemicals and low in bacteria. Glyphosate/weed killer for example
is great for killing weeds, and soil bacteria. Perhaps the farmers have

their hands in the soil much less these days. Droughts kill off plants and animals, but also soil bacteria too. Probably many, if not all the farmers, have taken multiple doses of antibiotics. Maybe, like the rest of us, they receive terrible news that the bank is foreclosing and the drought is set to continue, along with all sorts of other disasters…or their bacteria have been wiped out by antibiotics and they're eating the prescribed, modern diet and using sunscreen regularly. Or maybe their bodies can't cope because of all these factors, and the bacteria they receive from the soil just isn't enough.

Your Body is an Ecosystem

Your body is an ecosystem, and my point is that this ecosystem can influence your behaviour and cause Depression, if it becomes unhealthy. Look after your ecosystem and look after your bacteria.

Antibiotics vs Antimicrobials

Antibiotics, I like to think of as living things. In the simplest language they are moulds. Just like black mould that grows on your driveway, in your pool, or up the walls. Well not exactly, but close enough. Like all medicines, antibiotics are poisons. What they do is attack the cell walls of bacteria. The bacteria 'spills its guts' so to speak, and dies.

Antimicrobials on the other hand are poison chemicals that get inside the cell and kill the stuff inside. For example, chlorine, fluoride, sulphur dioxide and many food preservatives fall into this category.

The result is typically the same. Bacteria die. Antibiotics are just so much more powerful, that's all.

One last thought... if I'm right about antibiotics and the modern dietary recommendations (more about that later) as causes of Depression then the theory has a powerful, additional benefit. It alleviates the guilt aspect of Depression, which can be a huge relief for many people. You have followed your doctor's advice to use antibiotics and you have followed government dietary advice and those things have been a strong contributor to your Depression. That certainly takes a weight off your shoulders, but I'm putting it back on - sorry; now it's your responsibility to fix it, regardless of who may have caused it. Don't worry though, I hope to tell you how.

SPOOKY STORIES

- WHERE DO THE ANTIBIOTICS GO? -

Do you know where most antibiotics go? They're fed to farm animals, mostly cows and chickens. About 80 to 90% of all antibiotics used in the USA go to farm animals. Antibiotics are not necessarily used to aid the health of the animals. They are used as growth promoters. In other words, regular use of antibiotics make the cows grow fatter, faster. Could it be that regular use of antibiotics and antimicrobials is partly to blame for the obesity epidemic? Do antibiotics make people put on weight faster? My guess is…yes, they do.

- QUORUM SENSING -

Bacteria talk to each other and 'Quorum sensing' is one of the ways they do it. A Quorum means enough people to hold a meeting. You can't have a meeting until a Quorum is present, (enough people). It just means that bacteria wait until there are enough of them, before they start doing stuff. The first story I heard about this, was in relation to an octopus that glows purple at night. The glow is caused by bacteria. They live inside the octopus at night, but during the day, they live outside the creature. When outside the octopus, they're in low concentration, but inside, they're in high concentration. Once the numbers inside the octopus are high enough, they start glowing purple. So, if you agree that bacteria create serotonin, perhaps you need enough of them before it starts to happen. I am not saying all bacteria talk to all other bacteria. What they do is talk to bacteria that they like, or the others who are like them. When there are enough of them, they do good things for you.

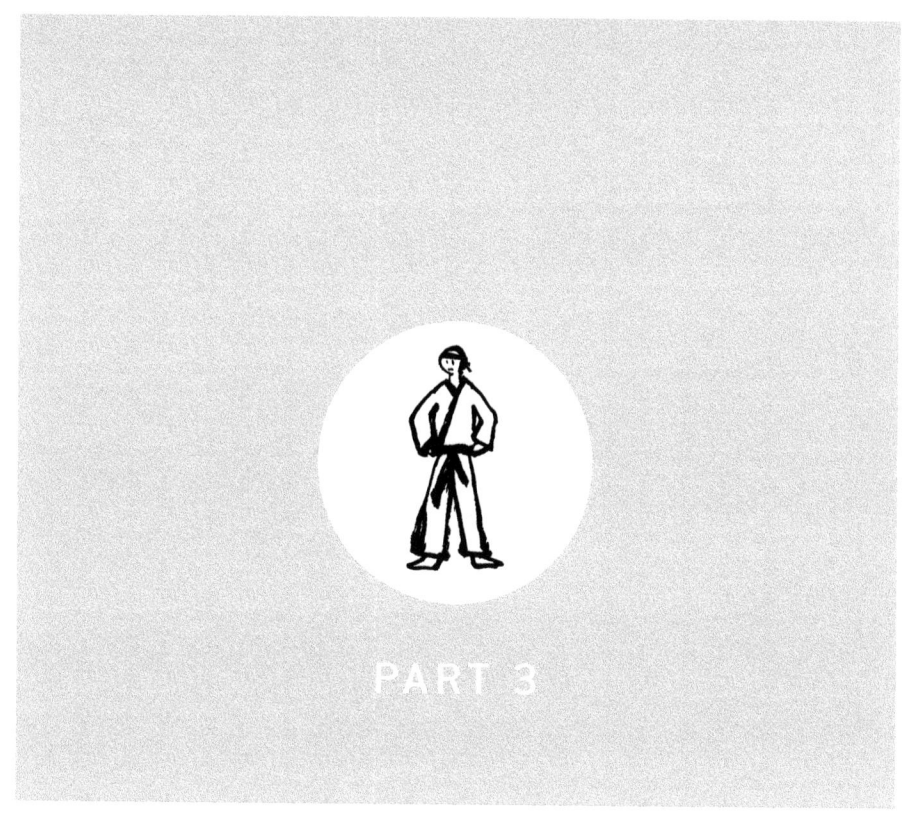

PART 3

FIX YOUR GUT!

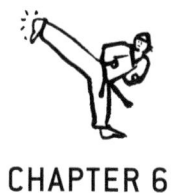

CHAPTER 6

Gut Health

Gut Health Summary

This chapter is a bit technical so if you don't want to read it, I don't blame you. It includes a talk I gave a few months ago on gut health; very poorly attended I must say, and I have no idea if my message got across. Anyway, I'll give you a quick summary here of what I am trying to say in relation to Depression and the gut.

It's my theory, and it has considerable backing. The Depression epidemic is largely a side effect of antibiotics. As I've said previously, don't get me wrong, I'm not against antibiotics, they are wonderful, life-saving drugs. Here's an article that backs up my assertions.

> *"Asking your doctor for another antibiotics' prescription? How just ONE course raises the risk of depression…*
>
> *Researchers at Tel Aviv University found that a single course of antibiotics boosts the risk of depression by around a quarter. Taking between two and five courses raises the risk by nearly half, they reported in the Journal of Clinical Psychiatry. Experts say disrupting gut bacteria harms the way brain cells communicate."*
>
> *(Web source: https://www.dailymail.co.uk/health/article-3605651/Asking-doctor-antibiotics-prescription-just-ONE-course-raises-risk-depression.html)*

What I'm suggesting is slightly different. Serotonin (the feel-good neurotransmitter) is made by bacteria that live in your gut. If you don't have enough good gut bacteria you may suffer from Depression.

What a lot of people won't understand is that:

1. Antibiotics kill bacteria;

2. Antibiotics kill good and bad bacteria;

3. There are a lot of good bacteria in your gut right now;

4. The more courses of antibiotics you've taken, the more good bacteria you've killed;

5. You can replace your good bacteria but it takes time, good food, and you have to stop ingesting things that damage bacteria, like chlorine and preservatives.

Anyway, back to the summary.

Now it's easy to think of the gut or colon/large intestine as just a waste disposal dump, but that would be a mistake. The colon, or gut, is basically your body's chemical factory. The gut is where many of your vitamins are manufactured, along with many other compounds that help your body function correctly. Your gut is just as important as your liver and kidneys, and almost as important as your brain and your heart. In fact, your gut is often referred to today as 'your <u>second brain</u>', but I digress.

So your gut is basically like a pipe; around 75mm in diameter and 5 feet long (as opposed to the small intestine at 25mm diameter and 6 feet in length). It winds all around your abdomen. But apart from the size and length of the small and large intestine, there's one huge difference between the two. Your gut is home to trillions of bacteria. Now when I say trillions, I mean 100 trillion. That's 100 followed by twelve zeros. It's a big number.

You can hold a million grains of sand in your hands, if you have large hands.

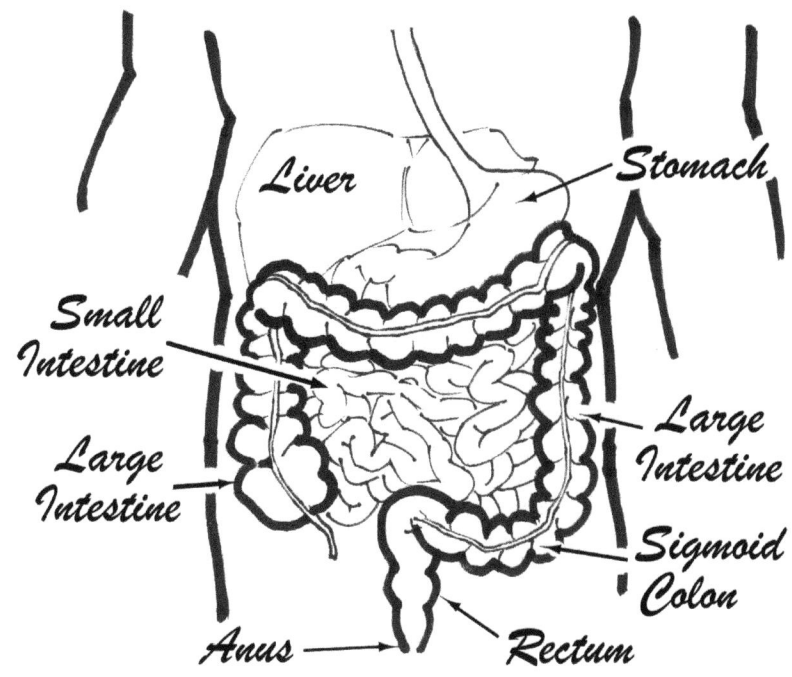

So a trillion is a million handfuls of sand. 100 trillion is the total number of sand grains on a beach that's one mile long, by two metres deep.

To put another perspective on it, your body is made up of around ten trillion cells. So, your bacterial cells outnumber your human cells.

A few years ago, scientists mapped the human genome. That is, they found all of the genes that make us human. Turns out we have surprisingly few genes, about 20,000 (more or less). Genes, as you know, are like building blocks or messages that build us; they make our eyes blue or green, our hair blonde or black, and our skin dark or light.

People often say, "It's in my genes," or "I'm wired that way," or "it's in my DNA."

Well it so happens that our bacteria have genes too. Each species of bacteria has about 3000 genes. So, if there are 1000 species of bacteria in your gut, then there are three million bacterial genes in your gut. And there are 150 bacterial genes for every one of your human genes. We are in fact made up of way more bacterial genes than human genes.

But the weight of all these bacteria is only about 2kg (5lbs), so obviously they're pretty small.

Just another little fact for you: 1 gram of your faeces contains around one million bacteria. (These figures sourced from UNICEF and WHO.)

Fixing your Gut Health

The easiest way to fix your gut health in my opinion is by way of probiotics. You can take many different strains, in different ways. These include probiotic foods like Kombucha and Sauerkraut. There are also supplements to soothe and repair your gut, as well as prebiotics (fibre) to feed your good gut bacteria.

My Gut Health Talk

This is a talk I gave back in 2018. I decided to throw it in this book (with little modification) because I feel it tells a good story. You will have already read much of this in the previous section and chapters, but as I said earlier, that was just a summary for those of you who don't want to wade through this. So beware, I'll be repeating myself here, and if you choose to read on, you also must forgive me.

• • • • • • • • • • •

"Gut feelings, gut instinct, get to the guts of the issue, trust your gut, grizzly guts, pain in the arse, you give me the shits, I hate your guts…we've all heard or used these expressions, right? Well there's good reason for this relationship between the guts and your emotions, and I'm going to explain why. A lot of people think that

---

the gut or colon is just a food processing plant with a sewer at the end, but there's a lot more going on than you ever imagined.

If I get this right, it will make you richer, smarter, happier, and improve your health. And you thought this was just about gut health. Well brace yourselves.

What's the number one thing your body needs to do right now?

I mean besides things like, "get me outta here so I don't have to listen to this guy", or "get me to the pub so I can have a drink." That may be what your head wants to do, but your head isn't in control.

The number one thing your body wants to do right now, and always wants to do, is to SURVIVE.

Your body is a survival machine. Every living thing has the same purpose.

The number two thing that your body wants to do is procreate, just like every other living thing. Scientists call it survival of the species. I call it sex.

So, 'survival' is about food, and procreation is about sex. Everything else in life is a bonus.

This doesn't suggest that life has no meaning, or everything else makes you unhappy. It just means that everything else, apart from survival and sex, is fluff, as far as your body is concerned.

You might think, "Gee, there's a lot more to me than that - me, the person." It really doesn't matter to your body. In the end, your body is in control and all it wants is to survive (and procreate, a distant second).

Your body is a fantastic survival machine - possibly the ultimate survival machine. There are so many of us in the world, because human survival skills are so good. Your body and your brain are always trying to protect you and help you survive.

Your gut is instrumental in this survival process and I hope to show you how you can 'love your guts'.

The Hippocratic Oath

Who here has heard of doctors taking a Hippocratic oath?

The Hippocratic oath basically says: 'Do No Harm' and 'Use your skills as best you can to help and heal.'

The Hippocratic oath is named after Hippocrates (Hipocratees) who is considered the father of modern medicine; a Greek who lived 2500 years ago. A doctor if you like…the first medicine man to document things.

Hippocrates said, "ALL DISEASE BEGINS IN THE GUT," and to a large extent I agree with him. I mean we know a lot more about science and anatomy now than when Hippocrates was around. But we shouldn't ignore ancient wisdom either. So, let's just say that a lot of disease begins in the gut.

Hippocrates is also credited with another saying that you may have heard. "LET FOOD BE THY MEDICINE, AND MEDICINE BE THY FOOD."

Now these sayings should be viewed as guidance, not gospel, but I hope we all accept that good nutrition leads to better health.

Of course, when Hippocrates was around, he didn't have much choice when it came to medicines, so food was one of his only options.

Anyway, back to the gut. It is probably not what you think it is.

I want to lead you to the gut with a quick overview of the digestive system. Digestion starts in the mouth, you know, chewing and saliva, but let's skip that bit and go to the stomach.

The Stomach

Most people are familiar with the stomach; it's not the gut. The stomach is basically a hollow sack that partially fills with acid when the food comes in. The acid is hydrochloric acid, the same stuff that you use in your pool, or to clean metal and concrete. And this acid is strong. If you get it on your skin it will burn. But your stomach has a mucus lining (snot) which stops the acid from burning you. So the stomach has a pH of about 2.0. Whatever you do, don't allow stomach contents to touch your skin, it will burn you.

Just a word about pH (or acidity)…

pH, Acid, Alkalinity

At this point in the talk, should you feel like a quick nap or wish to zone out, now's your opportunity.

The stomach's purpose is basically to acidify food and protect you from bad bacteria, and to break the sugars and proteins into smaller bits to allow digestion to take place. The stomach is a protective organ, if anything bad gets past this baby, it may make you sick or even kill you.

I know that a lot of people are into alkaline water and an alkalising diet. I don't have a heap of experience with it, but my feeling is that it has no real value. If you start mucking about with the pH of the stomach, you're doing something pretty unnatural and you want to be careful. Almost all food tends to be on the acidic side and this is the natural order of things. Hey, I didn't make the rules.

After the food leaves the stomach it passes into the small intestine. This is not the gut either.

Small Intestine

The small intestine is where the proteins and sugars are broken down into amino acids and absorbed into the blood stream. This job is mostly taken care of by enzymes. An enzyme is basically a chemical catalyst, but let's just call it a chemical. So, the acidified food is pounded by muscles (let's call them hammers) and chemically treated to break the food into much tinier bits, so it can be absorbed into the cells and bloodstream. Sugars and starches are turned into glucose and proteins are turned into amino acids. This is what most of us call nutrition - the food processing centre where the calories are absorbed. After a few hours in the small intestine, the food, or what's left of it, passes into the large intestine. THIS IS THE GUT. Crikey… finally we've arrived at the real action.

Large Intestine/Colon

Now before we delve into the colon, I want to tell you a quick story: part tragedy, and part comedy. The tragedy is that the leading form of cancer death after lung cancer, is colon cancer. A way to prevent colon cancer is by screening or performing a colonoscopy. Men in particular, should have regular colonoscopies from the age of 50. Here's the comedy part. It's a story I read online somewhere.

"Colonoscopy Journal:

I called my friend Andy Sable, a gastroenterologist, to make an appointment for a colonoscopy.

A few days later, in his office, Andy showed me a colour diagram of the colon, a lengthy organ that appears to go all over the place, at one point passing briefly through Kansas City ...

Then Andy explained the colonoscopy procedure to me in a thorough, reassuring and patient manner.

I nodded thoughtfully, but I didn't really hear anything he said, because my brain was shrieking, 'HE'S GOING TO STICK A TUBE 17,000 FEET UP MY BEHIND!'

I left Andy's office with some written instructions, and a prescription for a product called 'MoviPrep,' which comes in a box large enough to hold a microwave oven.

I will discuss MoviPrep in detail later; for now suffice it to say that we must never allow it to fall into the hands of America's enemies. I spent the next several days productively sitting around being nervous.

Then, on the day before my colonoscopy, I began my preparation. In accordance with my instructions, I didn't eat any solid food that day; all I had was chicken broth, which is basically water, only with less flavour.

Then, in the evening, I took the MoviPrep. You mix two packets of powder together in a one-litre plastic jug, then you fill it with lukewarm water. (For those unfamiliar with the metric system, a litre is about 32 gallons).

Then you have to drink the whole jug. This takes about an hour, because MoviPrep tastes [and here I am being kind] like a mixture of goat spit and urinal cleanser with just a hint of lemon.

The instructions for MoviPrep, clearly written by somebody with a great sense of humour, state that after you drink it, 'a loose, watery bowel movement may result.'

This is kind of like saying that after you jump off your roof, you may experience contact with the ground.

MoviPrep is a nuclear laxative. I don't want to be too graphic, here, but, have you ever seen a space-shuttle launch? This is pretty much the MoviPrep experience, with you as the shuttle.

There are times when you wish the toilet had a seat belt. You spend several hours pretty much confined to the bathroom, spurting violently. You eliminate everything. And then, when you figure you must be totally empty, you have to drink another litre of MoviPrep, at which point, as far as I can tell, your bowels travel into the future and start eliminating food that you have not even eaten yet.

Andy was looking down at me and asking me how I felt. I felt excellent. I felt even more excellent when Andy told me that it was all over, and that my colon had passed with flying colours. I have never been prouder of an internal organ. Flowers would not be enough.

On the subject of Colonoscopies:

Colonoscopies are no joke, but these comments during the exam were quite humorous; a physician claimed that the following are actual comments made by his patients (predominately male) while he was performing their colonoscopies:

1. 'Take it easy, Doc. You're boldly going where no man has gone before!'
2. 'Find Amelia Earhart yet?'
3. 'Can you hear me NOW?'
4. 'Are we there yet? Are we there yet? Are we there yet?'
5. 'You know, in Arkansas , we're now legally married.'
6. 'Any sign of the trapped miners, Chief?'
7. 'You put your left hand in, you take your left hand out.'
8. 'Hey! Now I know how a Muppet feels!'
9. 'If your hand doesn't fit, you must quit!'
10. 'Hey Doc, let me know if you find my dignity.'
11. 'You used to be an executive at Enron, didn't you?'
12. 'God, now I know why I am not gay.'

And the best one of all:

13. 'Could you write a note to my wife saying that my head is not up there?'"

(Web source: https://www.allprodad.com/colonoscopy-journal/)

You'll have to trust me when I tell you that the newer methods of colonoscopies are gentler than that described above. When you reach fifty, in Australia, the government sends you out a kit for a free colonoscopy. You should do it.

Now it's easy to think of the gut or colon as just a waste disposal dump, but it is far from that. The colon or gut is basically your body's chemical factory. The gut is where many of your vitamins are manufactured, along with many other compounds that make your body function correctly.

Your gut is just as important as your liver, your kidneys, and almost as important as your brain and your heart. In fact, your gut is often referred to today as 'your second brain', but I digress.

So your gut is basically like a pipe; around 75mm in diameter and 5 feet long (as opposed to the small intestine at 25mm diameter and 6 feet in length). It winds all around your abdomen. But apart from the size and length of the small and large intestine, there's one huge difference between the two. Your gut is home to trillions of bacteria. Now when I say trillions, I mean 100 trillion. That's 100 followed by twelve zeros. It's a big number.

You can hold a million grains of sand in your hands, if you have large hands.

So a trillion is a million handfuls of sand. 100 trillion is the total amount of sand on my local beach at Maroochydore: 2 metres deep x 25 metres x 1 mile.

To put another perspective on it, your body is made up of around ten trillion cells. So, your bacterial cells outnumber your human cells by 10:1. I've heard stories lately that it's more like 3:1, or

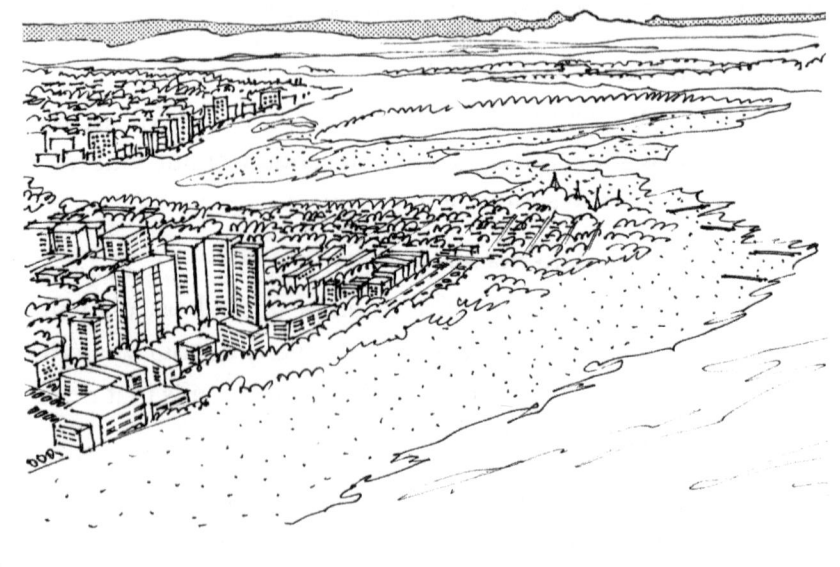

maybe 1:1. Whatever, it's still a huge number and bacterial cells still outnumber human cells. There are more bacterial cells on your hands right now, than there are people on the planet!

You are more Bacterial than you are Human

A few years ago, scientists mapped the human genome. That is, they found all of the genes that make us human. It turns out we have surprisingly few genes, about 20,000 (more or less). Genes, as you know, are like building blocks or messages that build us; they make our eyes blue or green, our hair blonde or black, and our skin dark or light.

Well it so happens that our bacteria have genes too. Each species of bacteria has about 3000 genes. So, if there are 1000 species of bacteria in your gut, then there are three million bacterial genes. And there are 150 bacterial genes for every one of your human genes. We are in fact made up of way more bacterial genes than we are of human genes.

Bacteria in the Gut

So, bacteria are tiny living things. Tiny animals if you like. They're everywhere - in the air, soil, water, on your skin, in your ears and eyes, in your mouth, under and on top of your nails...you name it. For the most part, they're good guys and are here to help; not always, but 'almost always'. You'd better learn to live with bacteria and look after them. They are not going away. The reason your colon (or gut) is so important is because 99.99% of all the bacteria on you, or in you, live in your gut. There are some in your small intestine and some on your skin, but those areas are merely bacterial deserts compared to your gut.

Just prior to birth we have very few bacteria, our own genes shape us, but we're colonised by bacteria during and after birth.

Bacterial Diversity

Let's accept that there are a thousand species of bacteria in your gut right now. Let's say these bacteria are animals, and they sort of are, like cows, donkeys, leopards, whales, butterflies, spiders, horses, crocodiles, snakes, birds, worms, dragonflies, and the list goes on. But it's even better than that; there are bald eagles, golden eagles and ospreys, hippos and pigmy hippos, Asian tigers, albino tigers and Sumatran tigers. There are also Poodles, Labradors, Great Danes, Terriers and Bulldogs. Now I've said before, your gut is like a rainforest or a coral reef. It's a very diverse ecosystem down there. I prefer to think of the bacteria as animals because there are plants too - but plants are more the fungi and yeasts. There are viruses and worms too, and most of them are also beneficial. We just don't know enough about them all yet.

Some bacteria are our friends, others we care little about, and some of them aren't that great. But on the whole, they all get along and are there to help us. Your colon, which contains the majority of your bacteria, is your own little chemical factory. It will produce almost all the vitamins you need. I mean your body can't make vitamin D, but that's supplied free from the sun. We've evolved to make what we need, and not to make what the environment provides for free.

I know I'm talking about your gut bacteria, but just to give you a general idea about bacteria numbers and diversity, let's have a look at the 'Human Belly Button Project.'

Belly Button Project/ Bacterial Diversity

In 2011, a sort of 'prank project' was undertaken at the University of North Carolina, but it eventually developed into a serious study.

Researchers aimed to identify species of bacteria in swabs of 70 belly buttons. Why the belly button? Because if you have an 'inny', it's one of the least washed parts of your skin. In fact, one subject hadn't washed in two years, apparently.

The average number of bacteria species in a person's belly button varied from 30 to 110, with the average number around 70.

They found 2500 different species, 1500 of which had never been identified before. They even found species on North Americans, previously only found in Japan. Those subjects had no connection to Japan whatsoever.

So, there are an awful lot of differences between us, and loads of bacteria everywhere. But honestly, the belly button probably contains only a few million bacteria. Again, a desert compared to the lush rainforest of your gut.

The general estimate is that 85% of bacteria living in our colon are good guys and 15% are bad guys. Who knows what the bad guys are doing there? Maybe they're just to stop the good guys from having too much fun and getting out of hand. Maybe they're the cops, we don't really know. All we do know is that the system works, so long as we don't interfere too much - which we do. We'll get to that.

Bacterial Species in your Gut

I'll just give you an example of the species of bacteria in your gut:

Lactobacillus Acidophilus	Good
Lactobacillus rhamnosus	Good
Bifidobacterium Longum	Good
Bifidobacterium Bifidus	Good
Streptococcus	Variable
Akkermansia muciniphilia	Good
Mycobacterium Vaccae	Good
E. coli	Mostly good (but bad E. coli can kill you)
Klebsiella Pneumoniae	Can kill you (but also makes vitamin b12, depends on the strain and the numbers
Helicobacterium Pylori	Don't know yet (causes ulcers if it overgrows, but also appears to have protective properties
Desulphomonus	Good
B. Thetaiotaomicron	Good
Clostridium difficile	Bad
Staphylococcus	Bad, generally
Salmonella	Bad

Food and Sex

Like every living thing, bacteria have only two real purposes in life - 1: to survive and, 2: to procreate. I know what you're thinking... it's food then sex, in that order. And it is. Everything else is really a bonus.

So most bacteria mean you no harm, even the irritating ones. It's in everybody's interest to keep you alive, because if you go, they all go. Occasionally an invader makes its way in, and it doesn't know the rules. Let's take cholera or the flu (a virus) for example. These guys are just here to party. The rest of the apartment block wants to go to sleep, or just go about their daily business, so they're not happy with the new kids on the block. The residents mount a defence and usually they win by outnumbering them, but it's also their determination and will to survive that keep the peace...lucky for us.

There are many, many beneficial things that our bacteria do for us, like manufacturing vitamin B12, keeping the joint clean, killing off the bad guys, manufacturing vitamin K, producing short chain fatty acids. They help with the stuff we can't do on our own, and they manufacture Serotonin. That's right, the feel-good neurotransmitter is made in your colon and 90% of all serotonin is found in your gut - not your head. If we don't feed the bacteria in our gut, we reduce the amount of serotonin substantially in our system and we suffer Depression. Now I mention this because my main gig is dealing with Depression and anxiety by improving your gut health. But for now we're just going to focus on your gut health for overall physical health, not your mental health. Though I would like to add in a bit about GABA or Gamma Amino Butyric Acid. GABA is the calming neurotransmitter. When you take Valium or Temazepam, or Roofies (like in 'The Hangover' movie), they work on the GABA system. They calm you down and take away your anxiety. You know, a 'chill pill' as they say. That's why Valium is addictive, because it chills you out. But you don't need Valium, you need to make your own Valium or GABA, and it's made by your gut bacteria.

Vagus Nerve

This nerve wanders through your body like a tree with branches. It's the body's communication superhighway, the internet of you, if you like. Absolutely everything is connected to everything else. But if you want to know how important the gut is, your gut has a ten-lane highway connected to the brain, in comparison to all the other organs, which only connect by a two-lane road, a dirt road, or a country lane. Apparently the messages between the gut and the brain are so important, that a major freeway is needed. The message is, that the brain and the gut are virtually one and the same. They want to know what the other is doing ALL THE TIME. If you believe in evolution, as I do, this means the relationship between the two is immensely important. If you believe in creationism (fair enough) then God made this superhighway for a reason. He wouldn't have made it unless it was important to have one.

I'm sure most of us are old enough to recall the bad old days, before the internet. We had computers, sure, and they were really useful, but I remember when I was a young engineer, it was only engineers and scientists (geeks) that regularly used computers; besides those typing up letters and spread sheets. It was the power of the internet that unleashed the true power of computers. Well your body, your brain, your gut, and the rest of your organs, are like small computers, all joined together. The biggest computers in your body are your brain and your gut, but it's the Vagus Nerve, or the internet of your body, that makes it so powerful. How you feel, how you react to life events around you … it's all governed by your gut, as much as it is by your head. Perhaps even more so by the gut, but we may never know the answer to that.

The Vagus Nerve is a Two-way Street

When the brain reacts to stress, serious stress, it sends signals to the gut. Likewise, when the gut is under stress, lack of calories, lack of fibre etc, the gut sends signals to the brain. It has been shown in studies that people with Depression and anxiety tend to have lower amounts of particular bacteria and lower overall diversity of bacteria. It isn't clear who initiates this: the brain, or the gut. That's why I often say that big life events can lead to Depression and anxiety. And on many occasions, after the event passes, the Depression still remains. The head affects the gut and vice versa.

You may be interested in this article: *Altered Fecal Microbiota Composition in Patients with Major Depressive Disorder.*
(Web source: https://pubmed.ncbi.nih.gov/25882912)

Sadly, you can't un-do the big events that led to your Depression. But aside from counselling, and the passing of time, you can learn how to process these events more effectively. What if there was an easier and faster way? I'm suggesting that the ideas in this book, in particular, the restoration of your gut bacteria, may well assist your emotional response to these difficult events, and improve your resilience.

So if you believe that there are 100 trillion bacteria in your gut, or at least there should be, then where did they come from? And how do we look after them?

Bacteria are Everywhere

As you now know, bacteria are like tiny animals and they're everywhere; in the air, water, on your food, surfaces in your kitchen, the outside of rocks and plants, on and in your pets.

Instead of ignoring or killing bacteria, it's better to learn to live with them, they're not going away, and without them we die. The 'good bacteria' in the world outnumber the 'bad' by many, who knows, it could be 100 times or 1000 times or a million times. The most important factor is that most of the bacteria in or on you now, are good. And they're great at fighting off the bad bacteria, and don't forget...99.99% of them live in your gut.

Where did they come from? Again, the answer is everywhere: the air, water, food, other people, even from our mothers when we were born.

If you make sourdough bread and leave some flour and water on the kitchen bench for a few hours, the mixture will start bubbling. The mixture has been infected, or colonised with bacteria and yeast that floats naturally in the air.

So again, if you believe that there are loads of beneficial bacteria in your gut, then you'd better feed them and stop killing them.

"What do they eat?" you ask. Without getting too technical, they basically eat leftovers. I'm not talking about three-day-old pizza, or last night's chicken nuggets, even if they had nutritional value, which they don't.

Fibre/Feeding Bacteria

Your bacteria eat what's left over, after the stomach and small intestine have done their job...which is hardly anything, especially given today's modern diet.

They eat fibre and special sugars. Fibre is basically complex carbohydrates which are long chain sugars, unable to be digested in the small intestine. Examples are inulin, oligosaccharides, wheat bran, oat bran, lignin (wood) and pectins (gels). The CSIRO and most other health organisations recommend 30 to 40g of fibre per day. Doesn't sound like much, if you consider a person eating 2kg of food per day, then fibre is only 2% of that diet by weight. But in reality, your diet is about 75% water anyway. So if you remove the moisture/water from food, which is between 40% for wheat, 95% for vegetables, and 75% for meat and fish. The fibre becomes 40g in 500g, or nearly 10% by dry weight. The CSIRO estimates that the average fibre intake per day in Australia is about 20g, or half of what is needed. My gut feeling is that for most people it is considerably less. So, the CSIRO recommends five servings of vegetables per day, largely for the fibre content, but they also recognise that 95% of people don't meet these targets, and that includes me.

Worse still, most of our fibre comes from wheat, corn, or grains, and they're mostly only the one type of fibre, called insoluble fibre. You need all types of fibre in your diet, including soluble, insoluble, pectins, inulins and lignins, to name a few.

So how do you do it? How do you get enough fibre? Well you could eat your 800g of vegetables, two pieces of fruit, and six slices of wholemeal bread, but you'll struggle to do this every day, or even occasionally. In my opinion, the easiest and most convenient source is fibre supplements. Now as you know, I'm all for whole foods and not too fussed on most supplements, but with fibre it's different. I'll tell you why. There just aren't many natural, complete high fibre foods around today. Even a lettuce or tomato in this day and age, is a far cry from the natural variety that was grown a hundred years ago. When agriculturalists change food or breed new types of food, often the first thing to go is the fibre, the second thing is the vitamins, and finally we lose the minerals. Many fibre supplements are made with the whole food i.e. chickpea flour or linseeds, which are very lightly processed, if at all. Fibre supplements also contain no additives, unlike vitamin tablets, which mostly consist of additives.

These supplements should be cheap and easy to obtain: slippery elm, apple pectin, linseeds, wheat bran, oat bran, chia seeds, and potato starch. I reckon you need about half a cup per day. Apparently it's best to start slowly, like one tablespoon per day, and then work your way up. Otherwise you get the farts, too much fibre, and not enough bacteria to break it down.

Forest Before and After Fire

Now if you recall, I not only accused you of starving your bacteria, but also killing them. All of you are guilty, and so am I. The biggest killer of your gut bacteria is antibiotics, which could be translated as anti-bacteria. That's what antibiotics do - they kill bacteria. They're great at killing bad bacteria, but they kill off the good ones too. This is unavoidable. The more antibiotics you take, the more bacteria you kill.

I think of antibiotics like an atomic bomb to your guts. Other people refer to it as napalm in a forest. Your gut should look like a forest, but after antibiotics, it resembles a forest devastated by fire. But a forest can regenerate, so too can your gut...and we will get to that.

Most people I know take antibiotics daily and my bet is that most of you do the same. Antibiotics are in your toothpaste, your hand sanitisers, and impregnated into plastics. They're in tile grouts, your sleeping pillows, in some carpets, some wall paints, and occasionally in your food. The most common chemicals (antibacterials) I come across are called Triclosan and Triclocarban. In the USA in 2017, Triclosan was banned from hand washing soaps and some cosmetics. Apparently, it's still okay to stick it in your mouth though. It's also still placed into toothpastes in the USA. Almost all food preservatives are not technically antibiotics, they're antibacterial, which is different. What they have in common is that they kill bacteria. Unlike broad spectrum antibiotics, antibacterials are not atomic bombs to your gut, but are more like scud missiles. They can be compared to a constant irritant like mosquitoes, whereas a snake bite is devastating.

Chlorine and fluoride are also antibacterial. That's largely why they're in your water, but they will kill whatever bacteria they can find.

Antibiotics

A single course of broad-spectrum antibiotics can easily kill half of your gut bacteria and half of the species of bacteria. Some of these species haven't even been discovered yet, and for others, we have no idea what they are supposed to do. As we haven't even identified them yet, they can't be replaced by probiotics. Some just naturally return by exposure to others, and the environment, but it's possible that some never return.

I know I'm painting a bleak picture, but in reality all that I'm saying is try to limit your exposure to antibiotics where you can, and feed your good bacteria.

Probiotics

Now I'm nearing the end of the talk, so I should mention probiotics. That could take an hour, but let's try for ten minutes. Probiotics are basically live bacteria. Usually probiotic tablets are bacteria in suspended animation. They're good, healthy bacteria, often isolated from people, animals, and sometimes plants.

Probiotics are great for helping restore bacteria to your gut, but they only come in very limited types. When I said you have a thousand species of bacteria in your gut, there would be fewer than a hundred species available in commercial probiotics. It's like this: Imagine the diversity of the rainforest. Commercially available probiotics would be like dogs, any kind, cats of any kind, monkeys of all kinds, then maybe the odd insect or two. All of these animals and insects have been grown in a laboratory, so they're not adapted to the rainforest.

Given another fifty years, we may get closer to say five hundred different genus of bacteria, but I doubt it. Some of the bacteria in your gut haven't even been identified. We don't know what many of them do, or know how to culture or propagate them. Then there's the problem of storage and distribution. Having said that, I think probiotics are very beneficial, but the best probiotics are the ones you already have in your gut, even if they're just limping along.

The two most common varieties of probiotics come from the lactobacillus family, and the Bifidobacteria family. The Rolls Royce is E. coli - but it's expensive and hard to find.

In my opinion, Bifidobacteria are the most important. The reason I say this comes from my own experience, and a study conducted in Japan, whereby 100% of babies were colonised by Bifidobacteria within seven days of birth.

The other thing; there's a human bacterial diversity project going on right now. I can guarantee you that every person who has submitted a sample (there are millions) hosts Bifidobacteria and all have E. coli.

Lactobacillus

Almost every probiotic formula includes Lactobacillus acidophilus. It's a great, adaptable organism, but actually non-essential. Only around half the world's population carries Lactobacillus, and the vast majority (almost 90%) are Caucasian. Because Asians possess far fewer Lactobacillus, they don't really like milk.

Lactobacillus is good for culturing and digesting milk, so it's used to make yoghurts and kefir. The problem with yoghurt as a probiotic is:

1. High sugar content
2. Low bacterial content

Consider the television advertisement for 'Inner Health Plus'. It states, "you would have to eat 22 tubs of yoghurt, just to get as many bacteria as one inner health capsule."

So numbers are important, but not everything. If one capsule contains fifty billion CFU (bacteria), and remember there are 100 trillion bacteria in your gut...then 50,000,000,000 (50 billion) divided by 100,000,000,000,000 (100 trillion) = 1/2000 or 0.05%. I mean it's still a tiny amount.

I've personally taken tablets containing half a trillion organisms per day, for ten days, and it didn't bother my gut one bit. I must say though, I was pretty chilled out, but in a good way. You could easily take 10x 50 billion CFU capsules per day with no noticeable, negative effects. I wouldn't start at that level, just try from one billion to fifty billion organisms and scale it up from there. That's not to say that you can't overdose on probiotics. I assume it's possible - but really this stuff is very safe. Overdosing is likely to give you a tummy upset, but that's about it. If you're going to choose a probiotic, buy one that has 5 to 100 billion organisms. Best to get it from the refrigerator, and get lots of Bifidobacteria.

Back to Lactobacillus…it's one of the friendliest probiotics around. Lactobacillus gets on well with all the other bacteria. It creates conditions that other good bacteria like. Lactobacillus is similar to the popular guy or girl at school. They get on with everyone. It's also very easy to culture, manufacture, and is adaptable to many situations. Lactobacillus comes in many different varieties too, just like most probiotics. For example: Lactobacillus Lactis, Lactobacillus acidophilous, Lactobacillus rhamnosous, and Lactobacillus casei. I'm not going to delve into all the 'purposes' of these strains here, but do a google search and you'll find some are anti inflammatory, some settle the gut, some chill you out, and some we don't know.

My Formula

The formula that I used to 'fix' my Depression was: 5 billion CFU (Colony forming units) prebiotics. They contained both Lactobacillus and bifidobacteria. It was a 'prescription only' product that must be refrigerated until use. There are many good probiotic supplements on the market. Start low dose on one tablet, if that does nothing, try two, then four. Make sure you add prebiotics to your health regime, even a little helps.

You're obviously better off absorbing your bacteria from nature, like the dirt, plants, animals, other people, natural water, clean air etc, but this isn't always easy in the modern world. By all means take a probiotic. I think they're wonderful, just get the best ones you can find, and get them from the fridge. Many unrefrigerated varieties are already dead when you buy them.

Now if you don't want to buy probiotics, you can make them yourself.

Traditional Probiotics

Make Sauerkraut (fermented cabbage leaves). It's a powerhouse of probiotics. There are likely more bacteria in one bottle of Sauerkraut than ten bottles of probiotics purchased from a store. It will cost less than a dollar to make, in comparison to $300 worth of supplements. But the numbers tell only part of the story. A lot of natural probiotics are destroyed in the highly acidic stomach environment, but some survive. The more of them, the greater chance that some will make it through. Sometimes, store purchased probiotics make it further down the gastrotract because of the capsule's coating. When you allow Sauerkraut to ferment, the natural bacteria flourish in these conditions and breed in huge numbers. The acids produced by the bacteria, and the salt, act as a natural preservative. All traditional cultures used some form of fermentation that allowed food (calories) to be preserved for the winter months when food would be scarce:

Vikings	Fermented fish
Europeans	Fermented milk to make kefir, cheese, and yoghurt
Koreans	Kimchi
Japanese	Soy sauce, miso, and natto
Indonesians	Tempeh
Indians	Lassi and yoghurt
Chinese	100-year-old eggs (buried eggs to ferment), tofu.

Tea and coffee are fermented drinks, but the bacteria are killed off in the boiling water.

Pickles were originally fermented vegetables, but can be artificially produced with vinegar.

Vinegar itself can be probiotic, if it's unpasteurised.

Salami is fermented meat, though much of today's salami is preserved with chemicals.

Before refrigeration and chemical preservatives, fermentation was pretty much the only way to store food for long periods, aside from salt preservation of course.

Making Sauerkraut is just about the easiest thing you could do in your kitchen. If you want to know how, look it up on the internet. It should be fermented for at least six weeks, but six months is preferable.

The History of Probiotic Medicines - Bloody Germans!

You just can't stop these guys. The Germans are always inventing things and giving us all the shits. I mean yes, they invented the motorcar, but if that wasn't enough, they had to produce the best ones, you know, Mercedes Benz, BMW, Porsche, Audi etc.

When it comes to wars, they've been occurring for thousands of years. But that wasn't good enough for the Germans. They invented really lengthy wars like the 'Thirty Years War' (1618 to 1648). Then it was time to step it up another notch, so they created the 'World War'. Because that experiment failed, they then instigated the 'Second World War' to see if that would work. It almost did.

My point is that the Germans also developed Microbiology (Metchinkoff) then formulated the world's first probiotic pill (during WWI), and the second probiotic during WWII. Just to be fair, Metchinkoff was Russian, but he studied and lived in Germany.

The point of this story is that the bloody Germans invented the world's first probiotic pill, and the second, and these pills are still around today.

Mutaflor

During the trench warfare in WWI, more German soldiers were dying from intestinal disorders than from bullets. Being at the forefront of microbiological research, obviously the Germans wanted to find a solution to this massive problem. It turned out they detected a special bacterium found in healthy soldiers that wasn't found in unhealthy soldiers. The Germans turned that bacteria into a pill and cured their intestinal problems; too late to win the war though, fortunately for the rest of us. That probiotic pill is called Mutaflor and is still sold today, one hundred years after its invention. Mutaflor is a form of E. coli. E. coli promotes the formation of serotonin. The first medicine that Hitler's evil, genius doctor gave him was Mutaflor to fix Hitler's gut issues. Without Mutaflor, WWII probably wouldn't have occurred.

Bacillus Subtilis

This was the second probiotic pill developed during WWII in Africa. Again, the Germans were losing much productivity to gut diseases. Poor gut health in soldiers threatened the German's superiority in North Africa. The main culprit: Food poisoning and poor water quality. The Germans sent a bunch of scientists out into the field to study the locals' diet and their gut health. One scientist observed a camel herder, scooping up some fresh camel dung and eating it. Horrified, he asked why. The herder told him, "That's what I do when I have an upset gut … eat camel shit, but it must be fresh." The Germans analysed the camel poo and found Bacillus Subtilis in it, a bacterium. They turned B.Subtilis into a pill and that solved most of their gut issues. They didn't win the war, but as I said before, they went very close. Bacillus Subtilis is also still sold today, particularly to aid travellers' gut problems, which have the potential to cause any sufferer significant gut distress, and mental distress.

Thanks Germans, for the probiotics, and the cars, they are useful. Just stop it with the wars, please? I'm allowed to say stuff like this because I actually like Germans, I may even understand them! This is due to the fact that my wife, and in-laws are all German and I can speak German. I've also visited their technical museum in Munich, numerous times, where I learned that the Germans invented just about everything. Sorry, I stand corrected … they actually invented everything.

If you delve into the history of many wars, you'll discover that keeping soldiers well fed and protected from diseases like Scurvy and Malaria played an important part in the outcome of those wars. Bacteria, parasites, and worms, are more important than you might think.

The Ultimate Probiotic – FMT

Faecal Microbial Transplants - my bet is that you've never heard of it. That makes sense. A faecal transplant involves taking someone else's poo and sticking it up your butt. Sounds sort of icky? It's actually performed thousands of times a year and one of the pioneers is a guy by the name of Borody, from Sydney. People come from all over the world to undergo this operation. Why?

Because his methods beat the diseases the patients have, more often than other treatments. Clostridium Difficile infection, for example, is caused by the overuse of antibiotics. It can be life altering, or life ending. At least 30,000 people die from Clostridium Difficile infection every year in the USA alone. A faecal transplant has a reasonable chance of healing the patient.

There's a centre in England called the Taymount Clinic. They have affiliates in three other countries and specialise in Faecal Transplants (FMT). Occasionally they save people's lives, especially from the antibiotic-caused C.Difficile infection. They've also experienced recoveries from Multiple Sclerosis and Depression using this technique. Research indicates that FMT has existed for thousands of years. It is documented in Ancient Egypt and also China.

So in brief summary, make sure that you look after your gut. Limit your exposure to antibiotics and feed your bacteria, live long, and prosper."

· · · · · · · · · · · ·

One Last Word...

If you're looking for something that gives you more confidence regarding my theory, for about $400, have yourself a gut test, like a Comprehensive Digestive Stool Analysis (CDSA). The test will reveal which gut bugs you have in your system, and where you're lacking, compared with the 'norm'. For my money, I'd prefer to go to the chemist, buy some probiotics for $50, see how I feel, and then consider taking the test. This science is only in its infancy, but I can confirm right now, if you're suffering with Depression, your gut is likely compromised; highly likely due to modern hygiene, the food supply, and antibiotics. But you can do something about it quite quickly. If you have the test, pay particular attention to the E. coli count. The good E. coli are scientifically proven to produce serotonin. E. coli feed mostly on meat and blood ... not your own flesh and blood, but ingested flesh and blood.

SPOOKY STORIES

- FMT -

In reasearching this book, I have read many stories about transplanting shit from animals to animals, humans to animals, and humans to humans.

Do your own research if you want, but heres a couple of stories I found:

- Transplanting mouse poo caused depressed mice to become more friendly and less anxious (mouse to mouse).

- Fat mice become thin when given bacteria from thin mice. Mice eat each others' shit by the way.

- A thin womens bacteria was given to her fat twin sister. The twin sister lost weight, even though maintaining the same diet.

- An Australian man, aged around fifty years, was treated for Clostridium Difficile infection using FMT. His infection cleared up, his depression disappeared, and his Multiple Sclerosis went away. His story was featured on *Sixty Minutes* (Australia) a few years back.

CHAPTER 7

Prebiotics

Bacteria need to eat too. Some of them may eat what you eat, but mostly they require fibre (Fiber), prebiotic fibre.

Prebiotics are basically food for the bacteria in the colon. I've read articles stating that prebiotics are likely more important than probiotics. I think the reason I cured my Depression so quickly is that the formula I took, contained both probiotics and prebiotics. Naturally, you need the bacteria in the first instance and then you need to feed them. The fact is that we all have many bacteria in our colons, but it's the makeup and numbers of those bacteria that are important. If you have a high sugar diet then you are feeding those bacteria (or yeasts) that like sugar. They are not the type of bacteria you're seeking in abundance. The good bacteria like to eat fibre (fiber), but don't rush out and get yourself a bunch of fibre, it doesn't work that way. If you suddenly start chugging down fibre to feed your bacteria, you'll find that you get the farts, because you don't have enough bacteria to eat it all. If you've been eating a low fibre diet (which is almost all of us) and you want to build up your fibre intake, then you should start slowly, and build up. If you search around the internet, the consensus seems to be 5g of fibre (as a supplement), so one teaspoon per day to begin with, and then build up. The recommended fibre intake is about 25 to 40g per day (Nutrition Australia, Australian Heart Foundation). Most of us will get some fibre from our diets. It's easy to get a small amount of fibre like 10 or 15g per day. It's just way easier not to get enough.

I remember back in the late 1970s when fibre was all the rage. Your body required fibre to keep your cholesterol down and maintain good bowel health. Everyone was running around eating oat bran muffins, bran flakes, and muesli was the new super food. They were right to a certain extent, but no one knew much about gut bacteria back then.

Let me define fibre (fiber) for you, because I know when I was a kid, I couldn't really get my head around it. I was always thinking about the fibre being similar to wood fibre, or cloth fibre, or fibreglass. Well they are all fibres, aren't they? Yes of course, but we're talking about 'dietary' fibre. Now dietary fibre is very much like the fibre in cloth or wood, you just can't always see it.

Let's take a look at wood fibre. Wood is actually a sugar called Cellulose. It's a very complex sugar. $C_6 H_{10} O_5$ is the chemical formula for cellulose/wood, and there are hundreds, or thousands of those units linked together. Humans don't have internal scissors to cut those sugars up, therefore wood is indigestible to us. Termites on the other hand, love wood. I guess they have the right type of gut bacteria or enzymes for the job. Termites digest the wood fibre and then fart it out in the form of methane gas. The major source of methane in the world (a potent greenhouse gas) is produced from termites' farting. You could cease all cattle production in the world, causing disaster for world nutrition and the environment, but the termites would still be farting out the majority of methane. Sorry, I'm digressing as usual...

Fibre for humans can appear woody as well, but often it doesn't at all. For us it's basically a complex chain of sugars (not table sugar) that is unable to be digested until it reaches our large intestine, where the bacteria are able to eat it. The bacteria then produce various beneficial things for us like organic acids, butyrate, and vitamins, but most importantly for sufferers of Depression - serotonin.

Wheat

Wheat contains fibre, but of course, the more refined the wheat, the less fibre it contains. In fact, wheat consists almost entirely of insoluble fibre. This isn't great for feeding bacteria. Insoluble fibre bulks up your stool (your poo) and attracts water. It's soluble fibre that feeds the bacteria. In the western world most people receive the majority of their fibre from wheat. A slice of white bread weighs 30g (one ounce) and contains 1.5g of fibre. Wholemeal bread (slice) weighing 30g will contain 2.5g of fibre. Now various estimates I see indicate that we need about 40g of fibre per day, or 14 slices of wholemeal bread (25 slices of white bread). Hold on - not so fast. Firstly, the wheat contains mostly one kind of fibre, (insoluble fibre) so it will only contain food for one group of bacteria. If you're eating wheat regularly, you probably have plenty of those bacteria. Having said that, switching from white to wholemeal bread, is a good start to increase your fibre intake. Sorry readers, your mother was right again ... brown bread is better than white bread!

SPOOKY STORY

- WHEAT -

If you just want solutions, you don't have to read this, but it tells us something about the importance of fibre. This story comes from Dr Thomas O'Bryan, a brilliant immunologist:

Tom likes to take all his clients off wheat, but that's another story. Most people in the west, say USA, Australia, and Britain, obtain much of their fibre from wheat. Many people are now developing wheat allergies or intolerances, as you're probably aware. And you've heard of 'gluten free', it's everywhere. Some of these people are just faking it, but most aren't. At any rate, I'm not here to moralise on that issue. The vast majority are diagnosed with wheat intolerances when they're adults, after consuming bread for many years. The wheat is making them sick for whatever reason. I suspect it has to do with the new forms of dwarf wheat introduced around forty years ago.

SPOOKY STORY

- NAVIGATING THE GLUTEN-FREE BOOM: - THE DARK SIDE OF A GLUTEN FREE DIET

A study published online found that 40,000 people who'd stopped eating wheat, by the following year, increased their chances of dying from any cause by 75%. That seems ridiculous. They stop eating the thing they're told not to eat, and they have a much higher chance of dying! Why is this so? The theory/reason behind it seems to be that what little fibre they acquired from eating wheat (bread, pizza, bagels, muffins, cookies etc) wasn't replaced by another kind of fibre.

Let's say they were getting 20g/day of fibre whilst eating wheat, but they now drop down to 10g of fibre, no longer eating wheat. They're already starving, gut bacteria just give up the ghost. I hope you see how important fibre can be. Yes, wean off wheat if you must, but you have to replace the fibre in your diet. There are plenty of ways to increase fibre that don't involve the consumption of wheat.

(Web Source: https://www.frontiersin.org/articles/10.3389/fped.2019.00414/full)

Where's the Fibre?

We all get some fibre in our diets, so where does it come from?

The answer is fruit, vegetables, grains, and nuts. In other words, plants. There isn't much in meat or animal products, unless you eat the skin, the hair, and the stomach contents of the animal itself.

Now if you're eating wheat or other grains, you probably already have enough of that type of fibre. But you need the other types too. Try green vegetables like peas or broccoli. One cup of peas or broccoli contains around 7g of fibre. Potatoes (which are not a vegetable) probably consist of 2 to 3g per cup. Oranges 2g, orange juice 0g, prunes 2g each (that's why they make you go to the bathroom).

The following table is a typical day's diet, showing the fibre content.

The Department of Human Nutrition at Deakin University Australia, estimates the average person consumes around 20g of fibre per day.

Meal	Normal Fibre Diet	Low Fibre Diet
Breakfast 2 slices toast with eggs		3g
Museli	5g	
Morning Snack 2 Cookies	1g	1g
Lunch 4 slices white bread with cheese, lettuce	6g	
Big Mac and Fries		3g
Snack Orange	2g	
Blueberry Muffin		2g
Dinner Steak, potato, peas	10g	
Strawberries and Ice-cream	2g	
Meat Lovers Pizza		3g
Ice cream with sauce		0g
TOTAL	**24g**	**9g**

Of course, the more fast food you consume, the lower the amount of fibre. There's another point to consider here. In the diet shown above, a third, to a half of the total fibre intake comes from wheat. I'd suggest that in a typical diet <u>more than half</u> of the fibre comes from wheat or grains. So basically, we're starving our bacteria, except for those wheat fibre-loving bacteria. So how do we get more fibre into our diets, and/or feed our bacteria well?

There are plenty of good foods to eat, for example vegetables. Vegetables are full of fibre. Most health authorities in Australia recommend five cups of vegetables a day. That's close enough to 800g, or two pounds of veggies a day. The general estimates are that around 95% of people don't achieve that. Getting enough fibre is difficult. I admit that it's a problem with the modern diet. But not everyone suffers from Depression. If you do, its likely cause is low gut bacteria. There's also a high possibility that you're on a low fibre diet, therefore you're not feeding your good gut bacteria.

Let's see how we can achieve a higher fibre intake, without making it hard for ourselves. I'm not big on supplements (as you know), but I do make an exception when it comes to fibre, because it's so hard to deliver enough of it in the modern diet. Before contemplating supplements, how can you increase your fibre through food?

First step is to increase your vegetable intake. Your mother was right... eat your veggies, they're good for you. That being said, consuming 800g of veggies per day, as recommended, is difficult.

There is another way, or at least one other way through food, and it's called resistant starch (RS). This is starch that resists being digested until it reaches the colon. This will likely be one of the more difficult concepts you'll find in this book. If you cook a potato, or rice, or pasta, then it has very little resistant starch. The weird thing is though, if you leave potatoes, rice, or pasta to cool (for 8 hours) then their resistant starch increases substantially. So, the RS ability to feed your bacteria also increases considerably. Without getting 'techno' on you, when the starch cools down, its crystalline structure changes, making it indigestible in your upper colon, but digestible in the lower colon. Even weirder still, when it heats up again, it retains that structure. So provided you cool the pasta, rice, or potatoes down, for at least 8 hours, they become food for your bacteria.

In layman's terms, when you cook a potato, zero resistant starch. You cool the potato for 8 hours, lots of resistant starch (food for your bacteria). Cool the potato for 24 hours, even more resistant starch. Heat the potato once again, and it magically retains most of the resistant starch. By the way, I don't know if microwaving works, but I'm willing to believe it does. It has to do with the crystallisation process of the potato, as it cools. Once it crystallises in the correct way, it retains that crystal structure even if you reheat it. You don't have to eat cold potatoes, pasta, or rice, you just need to heat them, then let them cool again, to create resistant starch. I don't know if it works with other vegetables, but I'm willing to assume that it would.

The 'Work Around' for Carnivores

You may have heard of the 'Carnivore Diet', where you basically eat animal products only; meat, fish, eggs, chicken, milk, cheese, etc. I've tried it and it seems to work well, but this diet provides very little fibre. Many proponents of this diet report the alleviation of Depression and anxiety, which if true, makes me question the fibre hypothesis. I think I've figured a 'work around' for that. The primary benefit of fibre is to feed your good bacteria. I believe there are also other compounds in animal foods that feed bacteria. A good example is butyrate, which is contained in butter. Others include the connective tissue in animals like sinew, skin, and even hair. Today you can buy gelatin and collagen from animals in the form of protein, and I believe it helps feed the bacteria in your colon, just like fibre does. It simply feeds different bacteria, and it is well known that a carnivore's gut bacteria are vastly different to that of an omnivore. Both microbiomes are legitimate and sustainable. The point is, if you're on an omnivore or even vegetarian diet, then your bacteria will benefit from fibre. If you get onto the meat diet, or almost all-meat diet, your need for fibre will decrease, but you will need to feed your bacteria in other ways.

The carnivore diet is considered extreme by some people's measures, but I'd debate that it's quite normal. It certainly has credible scientific evidence that it works. Anyway, should you choose not to opt for the carnivore diet, and I suspect most people won't, then get plenty of fibre...your gut will love you for it.

Bone broth is a relatively new superfood. All the health gurus and naturopaths are extolling its virtues. The broth is basically made from the bones of any animal with small pieces of meat attached. It's boiled in water and salt for between 8 and 72 hours. There are a bunch of good ingredients in the marrow, including calcium and proteins that aren't available in the meat alone. Allegedly it's great for your gut health.

The area of prebiotics feeding probiotics is all reasonably new as far as science is concerned. There are many foods that feed beneficial gut bacteria. Butter, Omega 3 oils, and bone broth are just three examples.

Fibre Supplements

If you don't want to use food for your fibre, then there's another way - supplements. This is one of the few instances where I think supplements can be of benefit. There are lots of them available, they're cheap to purchase, and provide food for your bacteria.

Some examples are:

Slippery Elm Powder: Very cheap and manufactured from tree bark.

Apple Pectin: Is basically apple flesh that has been oxidised. You can make it yourself by leaving grated apple flesh out to dry.

Green Bananas or Green Banana Flour: When a banana turns yellow, the complex sugars turn into simple sugars. When it's green, it contains plenty of fibre. So 'yellow' means no fibre. It's easy to buy green banana flour today, especially if you live in Queensland.

Acacia Fibre: Basically ground-up roots of the acacia tree. It forms a complex sugar that feeds your gut bacteria.

Raw Honey: Contains many complex sugars that are not digested until they reach the colon. When you refine or heat the honey, many of those properties are lost.

Inulin: A concentrated extract of fruits and vegetables. It contains loads of complex sugars to feed your gut bacteria. I'm generally not in favour of concentrates, but it's really hard to eat 800g of veggies a day.

Unmodified Potato Starch: Also a good source of fibre. If you can get it, it's quite cheap and works well. Even better, eat cooked, and cooled potatoes.

The point is that fibre and complex sugars are important to feed your bacteria. Getting enough fibre is as important, if not more important, than getting good probiotics. Fibre feeds your good gut bacteria. It's something you should pay attention to.

If I were in the advice business, and I'm trying not to be, I'd get some FOS (fructo oligosaccharides), some Inulin (an extract of fruits and vegetables), oat bran, and unmodified potato starch, if you can find them. Psyllium husks are easily available (as fibre) but a bit harsh on the system, and perhaps some acacia fibre. You can't always simply take a probiotic tablet. Some of the bacteria aren't available in this form... you just need to feed the bacteria that you do have.

Hey, you probably recall from earlier in the book, that while I was writing it, I suffered a bout of Depression. I just couldn't figure out what was wrong. I felt ashamed and powerless. How could I be writing a book on Depression when I couldn't even fix my own (again)? Remember I told you about the All-meat diet…well I was on it for quite a while, and I knew it worked, but I was a little concerned about the low fibre content of this diet. When the results of my stool test came back, I could clearly see that I'd been starving my bacteria of fibre. Within a short time (days) I managed to get my fibre content back up, and I felt 90% better. So what will it cost you to up your fibre? Almost nothing. Eat some additional fibre and see what happens.

SPOOKY STORY

- PREBIOTICS -

Not all that long ago, human breast milk was analysed to discover the sugars it contained. I mean the most abundant sugar is lactose of course, and that's why I say that lactose intolerance at birth is impossible. Until very recently, one would die at birth from lactose intolerance. It turns out that human breast milk contains around 120 different sugars, but no one had any idea what their purpose was. We now know that many of the 'odd sugars' are food for the various bacteria normally found in a baby's gut. These are prebiotics for the baby. Nature is reasonably efficient, so it seems that these 'odd sugars' are there for a reason, and essential, just as prebiotics and fibre is for adults.

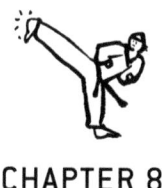

CHAPTER 8

Toxin Removal

In relation to anything that comes into your body: food, water, chemicals, or minerals, your body has three options: Burn it, store it, or excrete it. You burn sugar and fat for energy, but storing it means making it a part of yourself. Excretion means to dispose of it. Regardless of what the substance is, it must be dealt with. So good minerals, mainly salt and iron, become a part of you. As do useful proteins, fats, and vitamins. The bad minerals like mercury and aluminium, as we know, are cumulative metals. Yes, you can dispose of some of them, but it's tough. You can't rid your body of these chemicals nearly as fast as they come in, so they tend to accumulate. Chemicals like DDT and 245T are especially difficult to deal with, though it can be done.

The chemicals that you can't easily excrete are stored 'somewhere' within the body. One theory is that glyphosate (Round-up or weed killer) is stored in fatty tissue. This probably has something to do with the nature of the chemical, and whether it has an affinity for fat or water... who knows!

There are an awful lot of chemicals around these days, and they aren't always in artificial form. Natural chemicals like plant extracts can also be difficult for your body to handle. Large pelagic fish (Mackerel and Barracuda) can accumulate ciguatera. Ciguatera poisoning will make you very sick if you eat an infected fish. It's entirely natural though.

So toxin removal is carried out by a number of organs like the kidneys, or the liver. Until very recently in human evolution, there was only a limited array of 'natural chemicals' that your body had to contend with. Now, depending on your diet, there are thousands of chemicals around. Your liver and kidneys have adapted to help you rid yourself of these too, but organ evolution only occurs slowly.

There's another major organ that's also involved. It's your microbiome (the trillions of bacteria that live in your colon). The difference between you liver, kidneys, and microbiome, is the speed at which adaptation takes place. Bacteria breed at phenomenal rates and sometimes a new generation occurs within minutes. These 'new kids on the block' have to adapt to their new conditions. Sometimes the environment changes so rapidly, or with such strength, that adaptation is impossible. The bacteria simply die off, but if they don't, they adapt. It's like the saying, 'what doesn't kill you makes you stronger.' In some cases that's true, but not always.

When there are small oil spills, bacteria in the water eat up the oil. If it's a huge spill, the bacteria are overwhelmed, but eventually they do clean it up. I don't know if that type of bacteria lives in your gut, but your bacteria are able to achieve extensive toxin removal if they're healthy, and you allow them. That's where prebiotics help. Prebiotics are like food and fertiliser for your bacteria. Prebiotics can also act as a broom (so to speak), sweeping out unwanted 'things.'

The best prebiotic 'sweepers' are the harsher types, like psyllium husks and insoluble fibres.

When your dog feels ill, he/she will often eat grass to become ill, intentionally. This is an innate skill. In other words, this isn't something they were taught to do, it's an instinctive reaction. Usually it means that the dog has eaten something that doesn't agree with them. It's the equivalent to us being told to 'induce vomiting' if a person has swallowed some form of poison. Eating grass is what your dog does to 'induce vomiting.' The grass is an indigestible fibre to the animal. We don't know if it's fibre that the dog's seeking, or bacteria in the grass. But what may well be occurring is the bacteria in the dog's gut, telling it to eat the grass.

Aren't those bacteria clever little things?

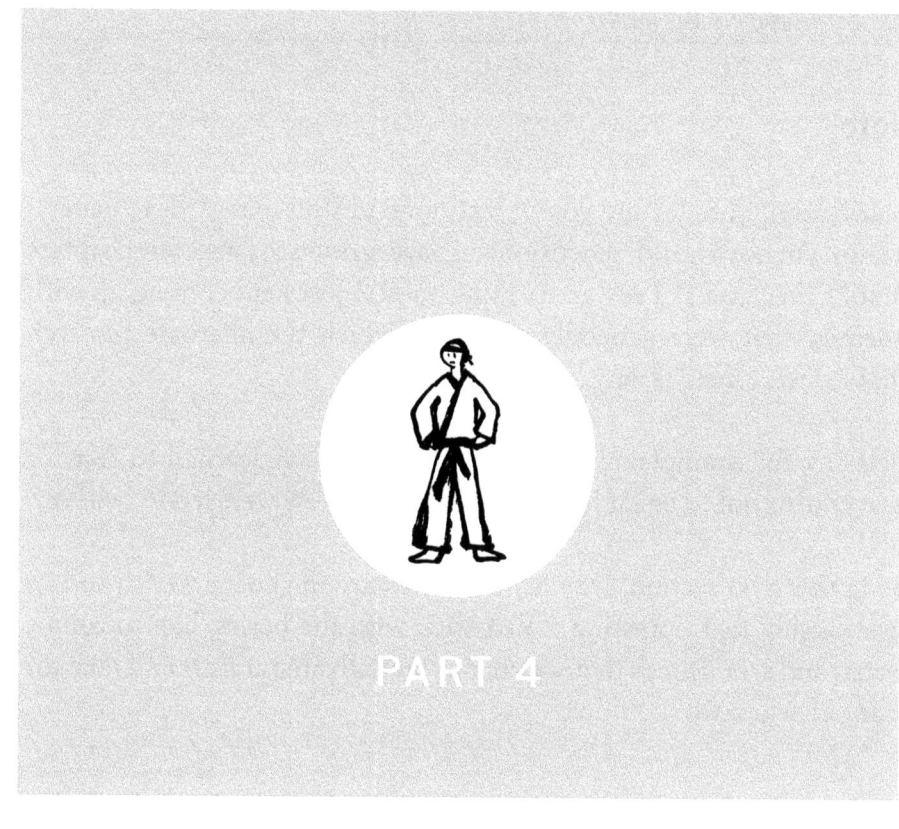

PART 4

GENERAL HEALTH

Note:

I have no right to lecture you or recommend stuff in regards to general health. I'm not a health practitioner. I have written the next few chapters though, because as I researched this book, I just kept coming up with 'themes' that were generally accepted, which the alternate research showed were dead wrong.

Lets say, for example, cholesterol; which we have learned to fear for years, turns out to be far less of a problem than we were led to believe.

So in this next section, I try my best to focus on general health and its relationship to Depression. I just stick with the basics, like sunshine, water, and salt. Things that we encounter daily in our lives and take for granted, when we shouldn't.

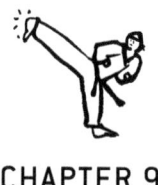

CHAPTER 9

The Importance of Sunshine

Let's start by saying sunshine is vitamin D. The sun and vitamin D, power everything in your life. I know that's a bold statement, but as far as I'm concerned it's dead on the money. So, let's go with the concept.

When you take a vitamin or any substance/chemical, there has to be a receptor for it. Like a key, the vitamin fits into a lock, which is the vitamin receptor. Vitamin A is good for the eyes and you'll find many of these vitamin A receptors in and around the eyes.

In regard to vitamin D, there are receptors in every cell of the body… every cell! It's the only vitamin that every single cell has a receptor for. The huge ball in the sky (the sun) has been shining down on us for billions of years, and it actually powers everything in our lives. The petrol you put in your car is like liquid sunshine. It is solar energy that has been stored for millions of years, and when we turn oil into petrol and burn it, we release that stored, solar energy. Sorry greenies… petrol is solar energy; it's just older and denser. I'm not saying that it's non-polluting, but it's still solar energy. Coal is ancient solar energy too.

A lot of people, including me, eat organic food these days. This means that the food is 'certified to be grown without the use of artificial chemicals'. There's probably a bit more to it than that, but let's just say it's 'as close to nature' as possible. The study of fuels and oils, and other carbon-based chemicals is called Organic Chemistry. So, petrol is actually an Organic chemical.

Maybe I'm getting off topic here, if so, I apologise. The sun powers everything. If you avoid the sun, you're doing yourself a dis-service. In terms of Depression, the sun, and more specifically 'blue light' and invisible 'ultraviolet rays', are accepted by the eye and cause serotonin to begin forming. As discussed earlier, serotonin is the 'feel good' neurotransmitter that's required to overcome Depression. Or conversely, a lack of serotonin makes you depressed. The single ingredient, and cheapest thing you can do to help overcome Depression, is to GET MORE SUNSHINE.

About seventy-five years ago when the Pharmaceutical industry was taking off, an awful lot of drugs were based on vitamin D. They just worked so well. Vitamin D was officially discovered around the 1930's. The initial problem for the Pharmaceutical industry: it was difficult to patent drugs based on Vitamin D. So, what the industry did was very clever, and lucrative. They set out to demonise vitamin D, because if they didn't, everyone would get well and they'd have no market for their medicines. Now that's not a sustainable business model. So, I'll give you an example of how it was done.

Almost all vitamins are measured in milligrams. It's a weight measurement calculated at 1/1000 grams, or one, one thousandth of a gram. So, for example, a large vitamin C tablet will be 1000mg, or 1 gram. For vitamin B3 it's 16mg. For B12 it's 0.5mg. The Recommended Daily Allowance (RDA) for most vitamins is measured in milligrams or micro grams. This is true of all vitamins except for D and E, which are measured in International Units (IU). I'm not going into detail about how IU is measured because it's a bit boring, but that's not the point. The point is that there are loads of them, IU's I mean. Only twenty minutes in the sun should produce about 20,000 IU of vitamin D. If vitamin D were measured in milligrams, then 20,000 IU would be 500mcg (micrograms) or 0.5 milligrams (half a milligram). So why don't we just say half a milligram? The reason…the number isn't scary enough. The pharmaceutical guys wanted to 'scare us' away from this vitamin D stuff by making the unit of measurement huge. Why? Because they knew how powerful and healthy vitamin D was. They made us feel afraid of the sun, in order to reduce our vitamin D intake. Then they limited the dose of vitamin D to 400 IU, a tiny amount, and encouraged people to stay out of the sun.

I wish this weren't true, and I know I'd have trouble proving it in court, but it is.

That brings me to the Eskimos. I believe they're known as the Inuit people, but I prefer the Eskimo reference. So how do these guys survive when the sun doesn't shine for six months of the year? Well, they eat their sunshine of course. That includes fish, whale meat, seal meat, and bear meat. If you look into these foods, you'll find they are loaded with vitamin D (liquid sunshine).

The world's most popular medicine/supplement up until about 1950 was Cod Liver Oil (CLO). That's liquid sunshine too, and it contains huge amounts of vitamin D. If you suffer from Depression and struggle to get enough sunshine, you could do far worse than take a desert spoon of cod liver oil each day. Hey, what harm is there in that? By the way, look up Wikipedia on the internet and search 'cod liver oil', you'll find some quality, scientific evidence of CLO being used as an anti-depressant.

CLO is also loaded with Omega 3 oils. If you still think that Depression's in your brain, and to some extent it is, then you might be interested in the fact that your brain is the fattiest organ in your body. 60% of your brain matter (after water is removed) is fat. About one third of that fat is a combination 1:1 of Omega 3 and Omega 6 fats. There are plenty of Omega 6 fats in today's diet, but very few Omega 3 fats. That means your body struggles to make your brain function efficiently, because it's not being supplied the oils that it needs. Oh, by the way my vegetarian friends, the omega 3 oils in plants and vegetables aren't the correct type (Alpha-Linoleic-Acid) and cannot easily be converted to the kind of

Omega 3 that your brain needs (EPA and DHA). Sorry.

The way I see it, Omega 3 oils are also liquid sunshine, and essential to good physical and mental health.

When it comes to sunshine, you have to receive it the way it's intended. That means no sunscreen. Sunscreen prevents vitamin D formation. I'm not saying 'never use sunscreen', but the aim is to get ten to twenty minutes per day of direct sunlight on your skin. This is the recommended amount from the Vitamin D Council.

Here's another little-known fact: Glasses, sunglasses, car windscreens and windows, block out 95% of UV rays. UV rays are invisible, but we know that they exist. So too do your eyes and your skin. If you receive light only through glass or plastic, you're filtering out much of the UV light. This light touches your skin, and with the aid of cholesterol, forms vitamin D that is used throughout the body. I mean it makes perfect sense from an evolutionary perspective.

This is a theory and I have no evidence to back this up, but if you filter out UV light, your brain doesn't receive the signals to produce serotonin. So if you don't get the signal, you don't produce enough serotonin, therefore you get depressed. I may be wrong, but I can live with that. Receive your sunshine in the way nature intended, not behind glass or plastic.

Not just Sunshine, but Blue Light and Invisible Light

Sunshine consists of natural light: all the colours, plus the invisible parts like Infra-Red (IR) and Ultra Violet (UV). Let's say even if they're invisible to the eye, they're still important. The particular one I want to consider is blue light, because it's so important to people who suffer from Depression.

Blue is the colour of the sky on a beautiful, clear day. In most places around the world where people live, this is normal, most of the time. The exception would be cities like Seattle, or London, perhaps the North Pole, and numerous places far from the equator. But for argument's sake, let's say that the 'normal' colour of the sky is blue…and has been that way for centuries (at least).

The blue light from the sky sends a signal to your brain almost like a direct order; it tells you that you should be awake, alert, on guard, and looking for your next meal. I'm assuming most of you would have heard about Circadian Rhythm, or the Sleep-Wake cycle. When you're awake for approximately 14 to 18 hours per day, the sun shines for the majority of that time and the sky is blue, most of the day. The blue light sends signals to your body to produce serotonin, the 'feel-good' neurotransmitter. When the light fades, it's a signal to slow the production of Serotonin and start to produce Melatonin instead. Melatonin is basically the 'sleep' neurotransmitter. Generally, it takes around two hours from the onset of darkness, for the Melatonin to peak, and this is when you go to sleep. The Melatonin generally keeps you asleep until the blue light resumes. It's production ceases at that time, and Serotonin begins again. The disruption of this cycle is known as 'jet lag'. If you've travelled long distances before, you'll be familiar with it. Your body clock has to reset to the new time zone. It also differs depending whether you travel west to east, or east to west, because you're either advancing the clock, or retarding it.

Anyway, jet lag is only one of many ways that your circadian rhythm can be disturbed, and this is important for people suffering Depression. Here's another good example. Electric light was only invented around a hundred years ago, so today we have numerous 'artificial suns' in our homes. They change the amount of light our eyes receive, extending the period of Serotonin production and reducing Melatonin production. The types of light bulbs we use are also important, because different bulbs produce different colours (in case you hadn't noticed), but your eyes notice the difference. The brighter and bluer the light (think fluorescent tubes and LED), the more blue light that's produced. Therefore, the more blue light, the longer the serotonin period is extended, and the shorter the Melatonin period. Hence why people sleep less today than they used to.

That's probably only half the story. The other half is that certain nutrients in your body get used up when you produce serotonin, rather than melatonin. You then risk those nutrients running out. I don't know which ones they are, but I'm sure someone does. So, if you're using up those nutrients, serotonin production has a hard time keeping up with demand. You become depleted of serotonin. As I said earlier, this depletion is what causes Depression. There's more to it still...blue light from your phone, television, and electric lights, don't possess all the wavelengths of natural light. We don't necessarily know the impact, but it must be confusing for a brain that has evolved over thousands of years, to receive natural light in a certain way. Your brain just doesn't know what to think of this artificial light source.

What's the number one source of artificial blue light production in people's lives today? Their mobile phones...closely followed by computer and television screens. The main difference between a mobile phone and a television screen, is the device's distance away from the eye. Basically, your body is being flooded with blue light all day, and all night. It's possible that if this occurs for too long, and you don't have the nutrients you need, you'll deplete your serotonin and experience Depression.

Now there are a couple of simple fixes for this. Fix No.1: Turn away from your phone, computer, television, and electric lights as often as you can. That's probably not a very sustainable model, but there is another way. Fix No.2: Wear 'blue light blocking glasses' at night. I've tried them and I can honestly say that the difference for me was fast, and profound. Instead of it taking an hour to fall asleep, it only took ten minutes. You simply wear the yellow (which blocks blue light) glasses for two hours before going to bed. Try it; you wake up feeling rested and ready for the day ahead. It's not a perfect system, but it helps.

You can buy yellow lenses for around $10 (maybe less), or you can purchase fancy ones for $100 or more. As long as they block blue light, they'll do the job. There are numerous books written on this subject, but I'll leave it with you to do your own research, if you're interested. I certainly hope that these suggestions can help with your Depression too. Remember... get plenty of good, blue light during the day, and lots of non-blue light at night.

Another thing: You can download an app for your phone or computer called F.Lux. At night it changes the colour of your screen to make it easier on your eyes. Makes a difference, especially if you're a heavy screen user.

By the way, when I mentioned Seattle earlier, I meant that it rains there all the time, so the sky isn't blue very often. This city has one of the highest rates of Depression-related deaths in the world, despite its very affluent standard of living. I see various statistics that suggest I'm wrong, and right - depends on how you measure these things.

Now I should say again, if you don't believe me about sunshine and vitamin D, and you're trying to solve a health problem like Depression, go and have your vitamin D level checked. In Australia, it's generally a free test, though they may charge, depending on where you live. The outcome: You don't just want to be near the bottom of the range for vitamin D, you want to aim for the top of the range if you want to feel healthy; like 100ng/ml.

If you aren't getting enough sunshine, eat it.

> *"Wearing sunscreen with a sun protection factor (SPF) of 30, reduces the production of vitamin D in the skin by 95%."*
>
> *(Web Source: https://www.catie.ca/en/treatmentupdate/treatmentupdate-185/nutrition/ overview-vitamin-sources-dosing-drug-interactions-toxi)*

Some statistics, showing the top 20 skin cancer countries in the world:

(Web Source: https://www.wcrf.org/dietandcancer/cancer-trends/skin-cancer-statistics)

Skin Cancer rates in Men

Australia had the highest rate of melanoma in men in 2018, followed by New Zealand.

Rank	*Country*	*Age-standardised rate per 100,000*
1	Australia	40.4
2	New Zealand	35.8
3	Norway	29.0
4	Netherlands	26.4
5	Sweden	23.5
6	Switzerland	23.4
7	Denmark	22.4
8	Germany	19.6
9	Luxembourg	18.1
10	Slovenia	18.0
11=	Belgium	16.2
11=	Finland	16.2
13=	Austria	15.0
13=	UK	15.0
15	US	14.9
16	France (metropolitan)	14.4
17	Italy	14.0
18	Ireland	13.6
19	Canada	13.4
20	Czech Republic	13.3

Skin Cancer rates in Women

Denmark had the highest rate of melanoma in women in 2018, followed by New Zealand.

Rank	*Country*	*Age-standardised rate per 100,000*
1	Denmark	33.1
2	New Zealand	31.1
3	Norway	30.7
4	Australia	27.5
5	Sweden	26.2
6	Netherlands	25.4
7	Germany	24.0
8	Belgium	23.9
9	Slovenia	19.7
10	Switzerland	19.5
11	Ireland	19.0
12	Finland	15.9
13	Luxembourg	15.4
14	UK	15.3
15	France (metropolitan)	12.9
16	Austria	12.6
17	Czech Republic	12.4
18=	Canada	11.7
18=	Iceland	11.7
20	Estonia	11.4
21=	Italy	11.0
21=	US	11.0
23	Greece	10.3
24	Hungary	10.1
25	Lithuania	9.0

Do you think that New Zealand, Norway, or Holland are places where the sun is so intense as to be a killer? There are way more arguments about sun exposure and its relationship to skin cancer than we have room to discuss. I mean try and avoid sunburn for sure, but get plenty of unprotected sun exposure when you can. Your skin is important to expose and so are your eyes.

If I had to pick one vitamin that is important to your mental health, above all other vitamins, it would be vitamin D, and the best source of vitamin D by a country mile is the sun.

SPOOKY STORY

- SUNSCREEN -

Sunscreen carries an SPF or Sun Protection Factor.

Where I live , the sun is quite strong and your unprotected skin will on average burn in 15 minutes in the summer sun (at approx. midday). That is called SPF 1. According to SPF theory, SPF 30 will have 30x the protective effect of your own skin. In other words 30x 15 minutes = 7.5 hours.

With SPF 50+ it's more than 12.5 hours. This is achieved with chemicals, mostly unnatural. I ask you...is that what you want to do to your skin? Is it necessary for your survival or health?

CHAPTER 10

Water and pH Acids

Before I launch into water, I just want to give a brief lesson for the non-scientists on pH. It's a measure of acidity. A pH of 7.0 is neutral, for example: pure distilled water. Anything below 7.0 is classified as acidic, and anything above 7.0 is alkaline. pH 6.0 is a weak acid and pH 8.0 is a weak base, or weakly alkaline. pH stands for 'Potential Hydrogen' but to most of us that's not important. The scale spans from 1 to 14 and it's not a straight line, but again that's not really important here.

pH 2.0 = Strong acid - e.g. hydrochloric acid
This is the pH of your stomach.
pH 3.5 = Mid range acid - e.g. soft drink
pH 3.5 = Mid range acid - e.g. wine or beer
pH 6.9 = Mildly acidic - e.g. tap water
pH 10.0 = Mid range alkaline - e.g. soap
pH 12.0 = Strong alkaline - e.g. caustic soda, drain cleaner.

People love ACID because our bodies love acids. Pretty much everything that you put in or on your body should be acidic.

Very few things that you eat or drink are alkaline (pH over 7.0).

By the way, you can't drink distilled/pure water, not for long anyway. It actually strips minerals from your body. This is well known and there's a warning label on the bottle. It's not so much a pH issue, as a mineral-stripping issue.

You eat proteins and fats, but proteins aren't proteins; they are actually a series of amino ACIDS. And fats are not fats; they are fatty ACIDS. DNA (your genes) is a shortened version of deoxyribonucleic ACID.

Below is a stylised graph of the pH scale and where foods lie on the graph. As one of my favourite philosophers says, (Dr Emmet Brown from *Back to the Future*)..."Sorry I didn't have a lot of time, so it's not to scale."

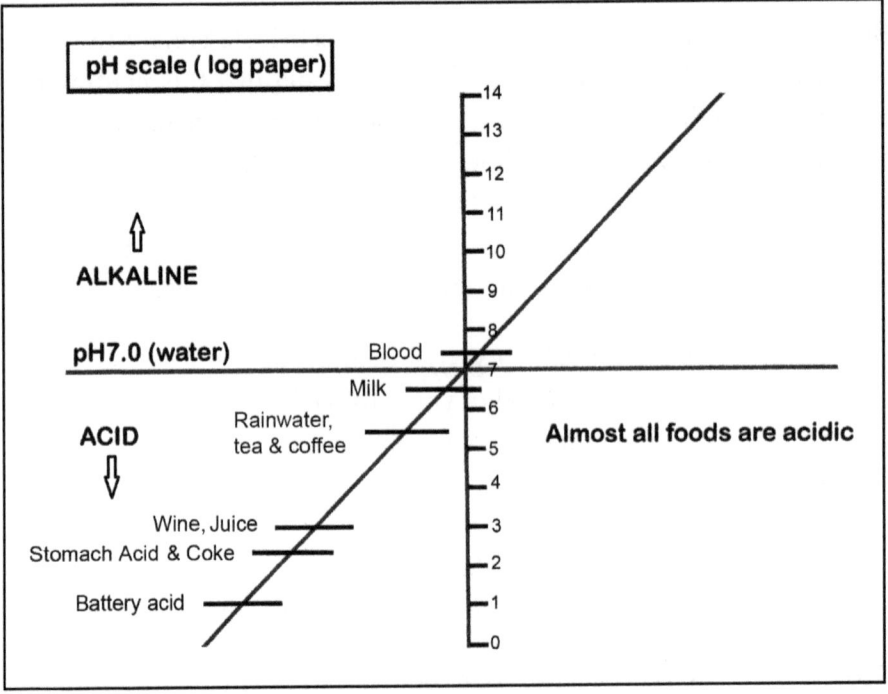

Your body craves acids. When you attempt to increase the pH in your body, your body fights back. When you drink high pH water for example (like pH 6.9), your body must fight back to lower the pH to what is comfortable. Digestion is made possible by hydrochloric acid in the stomach and bile acid in the gallbladder.

Gut bacteria produce loads of acid, e.g. lactobacillus will turn lactose into lactic acid. Not enough gut bacteria means not enough acid. And what about the wrong kind of gut bacteria? Well, the wrong type of acids are produced. Too much candida (bad yeast) will produce excess uric acid.

So, before I get into it, here are some fun facts about water. I should set up a table here to aid presentation, but hey... I think most people hate tables. Let's try this instead.

Pure water	=	pH 7.0
Tap water	=	pH 6.9
Rainwater	=	pH 5.5
Human skin	=	pH 5.5
Black coffee	=	pH 5.5
White tea	=	pH 5.5
Perrier water	=	pH 5.5

Rainwater is not pure. Water vapour is likely pure with a pH of 7, but the rain falls through gasses in the air/atmosphere and picks up nitrogen, oxygen, and carbon dioxide, which dissolve into the water. The carbon dioxide forms carbonic acid in the water, lowering the pH to 5.5.

Your skin has a pH of 5.5, spooky hey!

The world's best-known bottled water is Perrier. It has been sold for 150 years and has a pH of 5.5. People seem to like a slice of lemon with their water. There's nothing magical about the lemon, but citric acid in the lemon will lower the pH of the water.

The world's most popular drink, after water, is tea. Black tea has a pH around 5.3 and white tea has a pH of about 5.5. Adding milk to tea raises the pH. This is why many people drink white tea.

The next most popular drink is coffee. Black coffee has a pH around 5.5. Wine and beer have a lower pH; about 3.5. People just love acid.

The major part of your body that isn't acidic is your blood. This is actually pretty important. Your blood pH is only very mildly alkaline at about pH 7.4. The blood pH level is very tightly controlled in a narrow range. The message here is that the more alkaline things you put in or on your body, the more your body fights back to re-balance itself. If you use a lot of soap with a high pH, your skin will fight you to restore itself to its natural pH of 5.5. Also, the beneficial bacteria on your skin will die off at a high pH level and have to fight for survival to build their numbers up again.

Anyway, enough on that…here's the experiment. Try drinking water with a lower pH for one week. You could just squeeze in some lemon, or put in a slice. You could buy Perrier water, but dirty old soda water will do the trick. See how you feel after a week. I know this is speculation, but on the other hand, I'm trying to help you, to help your body and your bacteria fight off Depression. Every time you drink high pH water, your body will fight against you, just a little bit.

Strangely enough, this wasn't even the story I wanted to tell you. Here's the actual story, based on the interplay between water and salt.

It started in my head, with a question…something like this. "When should you drink water?" The answer is simple: when you're thirsty. I mean we know that cave boys weren't wandering around with water bottles in their loincloth pockets. They didn't even have pockets, or bottles, maybe they weren't wearing loincloths either. The only time they drank was when they could.

Anyway, thirst is a signal that you need water, or probably more importantly, that the salt level in your body is too high. When we drink, but aren't thirsty, we're diluting the salt below where our body wants it to be. Now obviously it can't always be in perfect harmony, but if we drink water when we get up in the morning, and drink a lot of it, regardless of whether we're thirsty or not, then we're likely diluting the salt more than is really necessary.

I guess I'm saying…only drink when you're thirsty. Possibly, some amount of the excess weight people carry today is low salt and too much water. If the body has too much water it has to deal with it. There are probably two options here, wee it out, or store it.

When my mother died from water poisoning, this is what happened. Her body stored the excess water in her legs. They were terribly swollen for quite a while. It only occurred to me a week or so before she died that 'salt' was the answer. I gave her a low dose of salt, about ¾ of a teaspoon per day, and bathed her feet in salt water. In one day, the swelling in her legs was considerably reduced. And, the leg that was bathed the longest, returned to normal in that one day, after being swollen for months. I didn't know why at the time, but I do now. The reason the water went to her legs was because her body was trying to protect its organs and retain its salt supplies. Too much water and not enough salt; to maintain the salt balance, her body had to dispose of the water somewhere. The legs are the logical choice for two reasons: gravity does most of the work, and there are no vital organs there. In fact, the excess water problem was so bad for her that she was actually leaking water from her legs. At least one litre of water would be expelled from her legs every day! Her body was crying out for salt. When salt is very low, your kidneys resist urination because a little salt will also be lost in the process.

If water is in excess, the body must deal with it, either store it, or excrete it…but it must be dealt with.

When athletes become delirious nearing the end of a marathon, it isn't usually due to a lack of water. The condition is called Hyponatremia, which is a lack of sodium, or salt. Sometimes it's called water poisoning. When you sweat, you sweat out a lot of salt. Next time you sweat, taste the sweat and notice how salty it is. Marathon athletes lose quite a bit of water when they sweat, but they lose proportionately more salt than water. Drinking copious amounts of water further dilutes the salt, until it reaches dangerously low levels and the electrical signals can't get through. Water and salt are the means by which signals are transported around the body. Pure water doesn't conduct electricity, but salt water does. Ever heard of an electrolyte drink? The salt is where the action is.

When it comes to marathon running, biking, or any high-endurance sport, our bodies aren't really designed to do these things; they're sort of un-natural. I'm not saying 'stop doing these sports', I mean I kitesurf, and that wasn't big with the cavemen either. I'm just saying that if you participate in endurance sports then water is important, but don't forget the salt.

If you go to hospital, they often give you a saline drip. It's salty water because your blood cannot handle pure water. Here's something else that's spooky... I just found out. What's the pH of a saline drip in hospital? It's pH 5.5! The salt content is 0.9%, which is the salt concentration that your blood should be. So, when they treat Hyponatremia in hospital, they either administer salt tablets, or they use a 3% salt solution and minimal water, like 100ml, three times per day I think. In other words, restrict the water and load up the salt.

All I'm saying is that you should pay attention to the quality and quantity of your drinking water. I don't profess to know the answer to this problem, but when billions of people drink water (tea and coffee) at pH 5.5; when hospitals hydrate you with pH 5.5; when rain is pH 5.5, maybe there's something to it. You will have to do your own investigation.

Whenever possible drink rain water. If that isn't an option, filter out the chlorine and fluoride. Add a little lemon juice to your water. Only drink when you're thirsty or when you need to. Water is important, but so is salt.

Water and Depression

Now, what does water have to do with Depression? The simple answer would be, "I don't know", but if you want to solve your Depression issues, you should give your body the best chance to help you do it.

Be careful of your water supply and aim to get the best water you can. Make it rainwater wherever possible, but that's usually not an option.

Filter your water to reduce chlorine and fluoride. (Chlorine and fluoride kill off gut bacteria). Note: Fluoride may be good for your teeth but there are no teeth in your gut! Fluoride should be topical, not ingested.

Add lemon juice to your water, just a few drops can reduce the pH, and you'll notice that it's more refreshing.

As I said before, salt water is a good conductor of electricity. When you dilute the salt and increase water, the electrical signals in the body slow down. This is because it's harder for the messages to get through. An extreme example is the athletes I spoke of earlier, becoming delirious because their water is too high and salt is too low. What if this was happening to you every day, but on a less noticeable level?

Of course, stay hydrated, but don't overdo it … and 'pass the salt' please.

Hot Water

Hot water, as a commodity, has only been around for about 70 years.

When I say a commodity, I mean something that's cheaply and readily available to the majority of us. Hot water is available on tap, literally, and delivered to our showers on demand.

Now if we take human history, and I'm guessing humans have been around for 150,000 years, then 70 years is a pretty short time in comparison. 'The blink of an eye' as they say.

So, most people I know (not me) have at least one hot shower per day. Is this good for us, or not? Where is the randomised double-blinded study? It has never been done … but we all accept hot water showers like it's our birthright. It's a bit like the refrigerator, or a car. Showers have only been around for 70 years or less, but we all accept and use them daily. This again is an experiment. We don't know if daily hot showers are good for us.

So back to hot water; I think ancient civilisations drank hot drinks. They possibly took occasional baths (like the Romans), maybe even frequently if they were rich. But hot water? Hardly ever I'd assume.

In reality, this hot water thing is an experiment. We have no idea if it's a good, or bad thing. Well I can say this, it's way more preferable than a cold bath or shower from a pleasure perspective, but what is the correct temperature? If I had to guess I'd say it's about 37 to 40 degrees Celsius, because that's neutral to the body. If you do a google search, that's what it comes up with. Correct shower temperature is about 37 to 41 degrees. I certainly know I've been doing it wrong for years. I reckon my preferred temperature is closer to 50 degrees.

When you wash daily, you take away dirt, salt, and oils from your skin...and bacteria (good and bad bacteria, but mostly good). The salt, oil, and bacteria have to be replenished. The dirt doesn't. This is probably why moisturiser needs to be applied all the time, because all the natural oils are washed away. Now most people I know aren't that dirty or sweaty from a typical day's activities, so why do they need these constant showers? They probably don't.

SPOOKY STORY

- NO POO -

I recently read about the 'no poo' movement. These people don't use shampoo. A new book is coming out this year called *Clean* by James Hamblin. This guy hasn't showered for four years. He only rinses with clean water every few days. You go through a smelly period, while your skin bacteria rebuilds, and then it settles. Once your skin bacteria are rebuilt, you don't need all those moisturisers and deodorants, but you will have to go through the stink period for a month or so.

Drinking Water

I don't mean the quality of drinking water, just the 'drinking' of the water.

If you cast your mind back 50,000 years or so, (still the blink of an eye), how do you think your ancestors drank water? Answer: They drank when they were thirsty, and when they could. They didn't all live near a stream either, although probably not far from one. They didn't have water bottles, or clay urns, and they didn't own water tanks. They'd simply cup their hands in the stream and drink. Maybe if they were really thirsty, they'd venture outside when it was raining and open their mouths. If they lived in Africa, they didn't go to the stream too often because of the crocodiles. Water was a rare commodity, even back then. They only drank when it was safe, and then possibly didn't drink again for a day or so. Today we drink water all the time. It's an experiment, and on evolutionary terms, a big one. We have no idea how this will turn out. I know everyone says stay hydrated for your health, but how do we know this is right? We don't. What we do know is that staying constantly hydrated is a wholly new concept. Becoming dehydrated or un-hydrated is bad…we know that. Does this mean that constantly throwing water down is a good thing?

The Australian aboriginals have been around for at least 50,000 years. As far as we know, they had no water storage devices. They were skinny and athletic, until the 'white man' turned up. I could say this about almost any traditional society to be fair.

Maybe, just maybe, the way we consume water is not the way were meant to. My advice, if I were in the advice business, would be to drink when you're thirsty, and drink when you can.

Obviously you don't want to die of thirst, but experiencing and enduring thirst for periods of time is quite a normal and healthy thing to do. I'd suggest it's good for your mental and physical wellbeing…otherwise you're ignoring history and evolution.

Water Poisoning

We touched on this earlier, but now we're going to dive a little deeper. Water Intoxication or Hyponatremia, is a latin word meaning 'lack of salt'. Natremia is sodium, as in sodium chloride. This is the chemical formula for common table salt.

Today, many Australians travel to New Guinea to walk the Kokoda Trail.

Kokoda was famously trekked by Australian troops during the Second World War. It's an arduous and perilous journey. I believe it takes about ten days to complete in favourable conditions. It's hot, and very humid. Still today, men and women die during this journey to retrace their ancestor's steps. One of the causes of death is Water Intoxication or Hyponatremia. Some of the walkers will consume between ten and fifteen litres of water per day. The reasons: (1) They're used to satisfying their thirst. (2) The conditions are so hot and humid. (3) They've been indoctrinated with the hydration message. But they have to keep the salt/water balance within a narrow range, otherwise they become ill, or die. In fact, the salt is much more important than water. Water Intoxication is what causes marathon runners to become delirious around the 15 to 20 mile mark, as we discussed previously. First the delirium kicks in, then they make poor decisions, drink more water, and if they keep going, they die. Think of your body as a huge electrical circuit board. The signals in your body are transmitted through your system as electrical signals. I mean literally, electrical signals. It's just that the wires happen to be your nerves. Water doesn't conduct (transfer) electricity well, but salty water does. So, when water levels are high, and salt is low, the electrical signals falter.

> "Exercise-associated Hyponatraemia on the Kokoda Track
> EAH is a modern, life-threatening condition which is preventable
> through adherence to sensible fluid intake during prolonged exercise.
> Although American sports and military bodies have revised their
> guidelines, researchers have been critical of the sports-drink industry's

role in perpetuating a culture of overhydration."

(Web source: https://www.mja.com.au/journal/2011/194/5/exercise-associated-hyponatraemia-kokoda-track)

And this from *The Sydney Morning Herald*: March 6, 2011.

"Media reports of deaths on the Kokoda Track often list dehydration as a suspected cause, but doctors have warned this could 'perpetuate a dangerous culture' when the exact opposite could be to blame.

Drinking too much water can lead to exercise-associated hyponatraemia (EAH) and hikers on the famous track were just as likely - if not more so - to suffer this potentially fatal condition, according to Melbourne-based Dr Eric Seal.

It was common for Kokoda's trekkers to start every day carrying more than four litres of water, he said, creating an 'environment of excess water' as they undertook the demanding hike in tropical heat.

'Well meaning guides and colleagues' could also encourage over-hydration while the early symptoms of EAH looked like heat exhaustion, and so could prompt even more fluid intake."

Dr Angie Hayes (BSc, PhD), a Biochemist/Nutritionist, in 2010 wrote:

"I was very surprised and deeply shocked watching '60 Minutes' today to hear that people actually die on the Kokoda Trail because they have not been taught about water and salt. I would have thought it was one of the most fundamental things to teach people doing physically demanding things in a hot climate: drink plenty of fluid but also keep up your electrolytes. There is a number of ways of doing this:

1. *Make sure to have a good salt content in your diet – some do gooders try to tell us that salt is bad for us but this originates from a very low percentage of people who get high blood pressure from salt – a very rare condition indeed. Salt restriction may cause you to drop dead now!*

2. *Add electrolytes like Staminade, Sports Plus, Isostar or even just some salt tablets to your drink rather than have pure water which will leach out all of your vital electrolytes.*

3. *Don't drink absolutely copious amounts, listen to your body rather than someone who may not know the full truth.*

Happy hiking!"

(Web source: https://kokodatrekkingaust.com.au/forums/topic/of-water-salt-and-death/)

So, I think it's possible that often in modern, rich countries like Australia, many people live in a state of mild water intoxication all the time.

Anyway, my analysis is that water isn't as safe and benign as most people would like to believe.

Now my wife quite reasonably points out that I may be straying into the area of general health here, and she has a good point. I guess in terms of Depression, I'm trying to say three things: (1) Don't believe everything you've been told about general health and water, just because everyone says it to be so. (2) I'm attempting to give you the best advice I can, to relieve this awful state of Depression. And (3) Even water isn't as safe as we're led to believe. Too much of a good thing, even water, can be a problem.

Ancient Water

Just some food for thought...a thousand years ago, where did our water come from? We got it, from a stream or a river. Unless we were really lucky (which was rare), the colour of this water would have been brownish, not clear. That was because the water carried soil, minerals and bacteria. It was an ancient version of mineral water. Of course, the mineral content was dependent on what soil or rocks the water flowed over, and where we lived. Now we drink water that is devoid of that high mineral content. If water comes from dams, then very little of it actually contacts the earth. Then it's purified, filtered, and chlorinated, usually resulting in a perfectly clear colour. I'm not complaining about it, just saying that it's very different, a vast change from the water of old. I mean I'd baulk at drinking water that was cloudy or muddy, as I suspect you would. I'm just suggesting that it's a massive change that we all accept, but it may not be ideal. I don't know the answer to that, but it's certainly a question worth asking.

If you're as old as me, you'll remember this scene from *Back to The Future 3*. Marty is sitting down to dinner with his Great Grandfather, the first 'McFly' in America. The water was brown and the rabbit had leadshot in it. Brownish coloured water was possibly the norm back then. That colour comes from somewhere or some-thing. I'm just saying that modern water is possibly nothing like ancient water.

Water Addendum

From everything I've read and researched, they state that the amount of drinking water you need to consume is two litres per day; slightly more or less, depending on size and gender. I'm prepared to accept that. Where I think the problem lies is a lack of electrolytes (minerals) in that water, and the pH. In other words, drinking too much 'pure water' may not be good for you. If you were drinking from a stream hundreds of years ago, you'd be picking up all sorts of minerals from the particular area in which you lived. Now we get traces of chlorine and fluoride, but it's really lacking in balanced minerals. Now I don't know what the healthiest water is, or the best mix of minerals. I just think it's possible that constantly drinking tap water with the same chemical content, day after day, probably isn't the healthiest thing you can consume. I'm guessing that two litres might be the correct amount, but at the very least it should be more mineral laden than your current intake.

Actually, here's something new for you...this drinking two litres per day, and the source of this water, has bothered me for a while. I recently read a book about fibre called *Fiber Menace*, and the answers came flooding in. Two litres per day is about right, but it's far more complicated than that. This amount is supposed to include water from all sources, but naturally, there are other sources to take into account. Thirst is primarily an evolutionary mechanism and secondly a learned response, as I mentioned. Let's deal with the actual amount of water the body needs and from where we obtain it.

Say we accept the quantity of two litres, even though there's no scientific evidence to back this up, but it's not unreasonable. The question is: Are there other sources of water besides drinking? The answer is yes. Food is the biggest contributor here, with most foods being in the range of 50 to 95% water (e.g dry meat 50%, watermelon 95%). Depending on the composition of your diet, water from food will add up to approximately 750ml per day.

But there's also a third source, and it's internally sourced. It's called oxidation water. This is a chemical by-product of the oxidative reactions that take place in the body every day, and it's in the order of around 350ml. In other words, chemical reactions take place in your body and water is the by-product. This means that the remaining water required (apart from food and oxidation) is about one litre.

So, as I said earlier, it's possible that a great deal of the additional weight carried by people is excess water. Not only does it add to your body mass, it also dilutes electrolytes (salts) and stresses the body and kidneys. I mean obviously if you drink coffee or wine for example, you'll also add extra water, because these beverages require water to flush out the 'toxins' (alcohol or caffeine) from your body. There needs to be an adjustment for the water consumed in these drinks. The same can be said for soda drinks, due to the sugar content. If you perspire a lot, you also need extra water. Point is...if you only drink water, have a normal diet and don't sweat much, then the right amount appears to be closer to 1000ml per day, not two litres of liquid water. Now I know this is heresy, but it could be worth a try. Maybe cut back to about a litre a day, and see what happens. Now if you're already hooked on water, you can't just cut back that much and expect a smooth ride. You have to ease yourself into it. If you're thirsty drink more – if not, don't drink anything.

And another thing, can you imagine cavemen running around drinking eight glasses of water per day? They only drank when they were thirsty and when they could. Their only receptacle was their hands, so they could only slurp up a few good handfuls at a time, then that was it for quite a while (unless they'd been out hunting or trekking for many miles). Even then, they most likely slurped up a litre or so and continued going about their business. They also wouldn't want a full belly of water in case something was eyeing them off for a meal.

I suspect a lot of us are deficient in all kinds of minerals today, because we don't drink mineralised water, or if we do, it's very high in some added minerals, but low in others. And, we're continually flushing minerals out of our systems by over-drinking water.

I admit this is new information to me and I haven't done the experiment to find out for myself. What I am saying though is beware of the suggestion to 'drink at least two litres of water a day'. It may not be what you need.

SPOOKY STORY

- ALCOHOL -

Beer and wine have been used for centuries as a preservative to keep drinking water 'drinkable'. Stored drinking water, especially on ships, can become quickly contaminated with bacteria or algae. Hundreds of years ago for example, Christopher Columbus aboard the ship *Santa Maria*, carried beer for his regular sailors. The ship was provisioned with the equivalent of one gallon of beer for each man, per day. More than likely, higher-ranking officers preferred wine. The massive content of yeast in this beer prevented the growth of other organisms, and the alcohol killed many bad bacteria, even in low concentrations. During the Cholera epidemic in Scotland, gin was promoted as a preventative to Cholera infections. Water mixed with gin was less likely to be contaminated with Cholera. Good, clean water is good for you. If it's not readily available, add a little alcohol, good bacteria, and salt to improve it.

CHAPTER 11

The Importance of Salt

In this chapter we are mostly talking about common, ordinary table salt.

NaCl = Sodium Chloride (salt)
Na = Sodium (Natrium in Latin or German)
Cl = Chloride (not the same as chlorine, but part of it).

1g salt = 0.4g Sodium
10g salt = 4g sodium

Almost all the salt in the ocean (85%) is Sodium Chloride: 10% is Magnesium Sulphate (Epsom Salts) and the remaining 5% is made up of other salts, dozens of them, like Potassium Chloride and Calcium Carbonate.

Salt, (NaCl) is extremely common on the earth's surface, and it makes evolutionary sense that it is important to our health. We may well have evolved in the ocean and gradually crawled out. I don't know, but it's possible. There are certainly many thriving communities near our oceans.

Salt is hugely important, and you should aim to consume around 10g per day (about two teaspoons). 10g seems to be the sweet spot. The average world salt intake of 7 billion people is about 10g per day. I'd back the judgement of these people over the doctors at WHO (World

Health Organisation) or The Heart Foundation, any day. I've seen estimates where Norwegians used to consume 100g of salt per day, with no apparent health defects, back before refrigeration was invented. You will see plenty of studies justifying a low salt intake. The WHO's own figures indicate that a salt consumption of 10g per day leads to the highest longevity.

This means 10g per day, corresponds with the highest life expectancy and the lowest level of cardiac disease. The salt intake recommendations from the American Heart Association, WHO, and NHS (U.K.) correspond with lower life expectancy and a higher incidence of heart disease. Additionally, the commentary is that 10g/day of salt is the norm for most people (people instinctively know this) and there's little chance of changing it; and no compelling reason to try.

GRAPH 1.

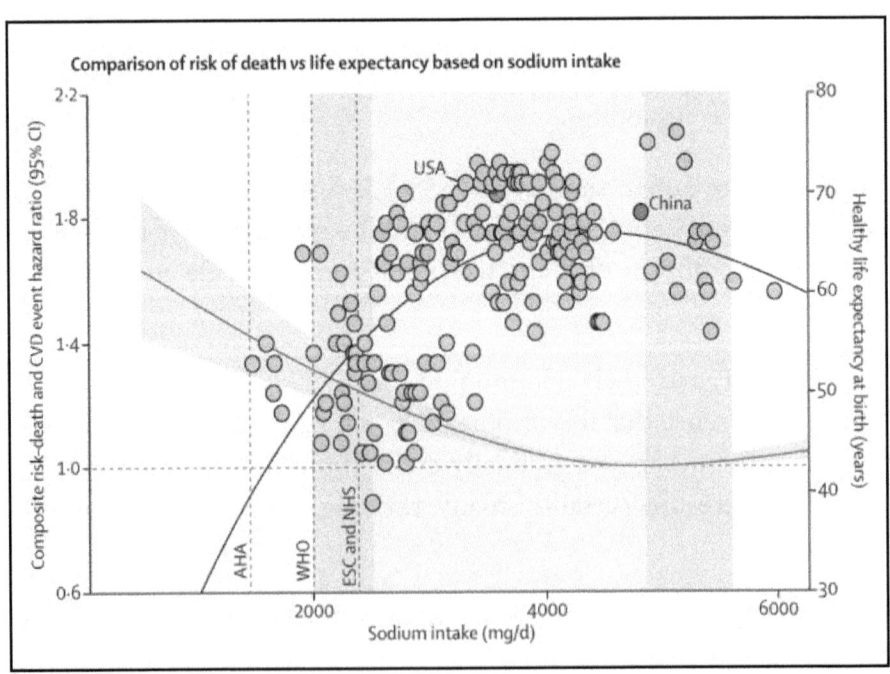

(Web Source: https://www.thelancet.com/journals/lancet/article/PIIS0140-6736(19)30232-6/fulltext)

There have been numerous large salt consumption studies conducted, with *Intersalt* being the largest. All recommendations arising from these studies have been the same: Keep your salt intake down to lower your blood pressure and reduce your risk of heart disease.

Unfortunately, this is not what the data actually indicates. The opposite is more likely true. Salt should be kept relatively high, with the sweet spot being around 11gms per day. Humans seem to instinctively know this, and the world average hovers around this number.

I'd like to explain these graphs, not in relation to Depression, but in this case, longevity and heart disease.

Graph 1 (opposite): Shows that life expectancy and salt consumption are closely linked. Sweet spot at 4g of sodium per day = 10g salt.

Graph 2 (below): It's a bit more complicated. The 'outliers included' line rises up as salt intake increases. This means the more salt that's

GRAPH 2.

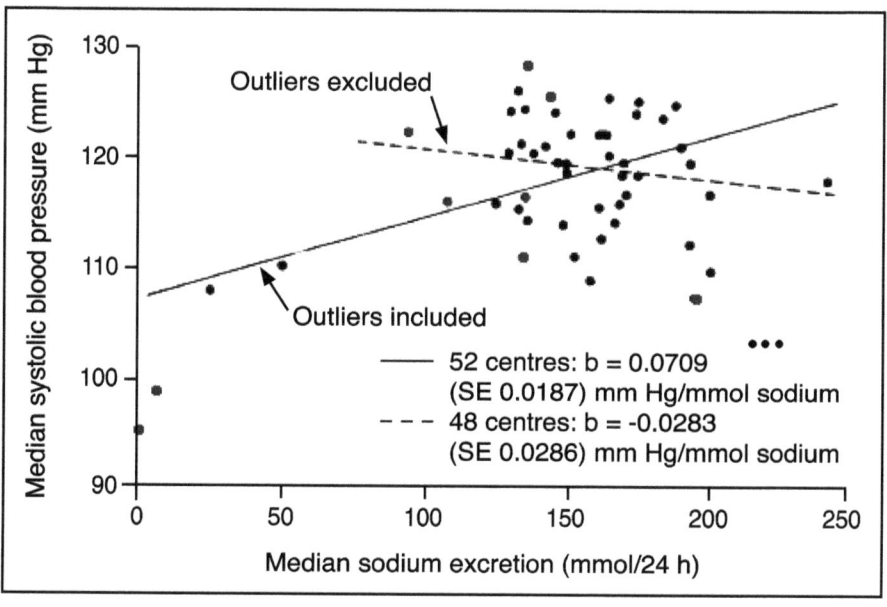

(Web source: https://medium.com/@drjasonfung/the-salt-scam-1973d73dccd)

consumed, the higher the blood pressure. The 'outliers excluded' line, is a far more interesting one...because it was introduced by others not involved in the Intersalt Study. Basically speaking, once three or more of the remote African, South American, and New Guinean tribes are excluded, the opposite effect is noted. More salt...and the blood pressure goes down. There are good reasons to exclude the outliers, which occurs in many studies. For example; these tribes don't have long life exptectancies, may easily have evolved from quite different genes, and their diets are vastly different from the rest of the world.

Let's just say that you or someone you know suffers from Depression, which is why you bought this book. We're going to concentrate on getting rid of it, and doing that as quickly as we can. Then if you decide to go back to all the crazy recommendations about salt made by the WHO and medical groups etc, so be it.

Apparently, they all want you to live to a hundred. I don't care about that, I just want your Depression gone. Having dined at the Depression table myself, I can tell you that living to a hundred with this condition would be more like dragging a chain with you all your life. I'd rather die at sixty, without Depression, any day.

When you take a blood test and they check for the IONS, it's called a Cumulative Serum Biochemistry Test. What are the first three findings published? The answer is Sodium, Potassium and Chloride. This is not organised in alphabetical order, like most things. It's delivered in order of <u>importance</u> ... well that's my theory anyway and I'm sticking with it.

Regular salt is mostly 95%+ Sodium and Chloride. NaCl is the chemical formula. Na = sodium because it's translated from German, where Sodium is called Natrium; hence the 'Na'.

Here are some recent lab tests of mine:

CUMULATIVE SERUM BIOCHEMISTRY

	09/10/15	14/03/16	28/04/17	28/05/18	
Date	09/10/15	14/03/16	28/04/17	28/05/18	
Time	13:40	07:35	08:46	10:15	
Lab No	61256282	72018412	64809570	59455156	
	FASTING	FASTING	RANDOM	FASTING	
FASTING					
Sodium	144	138	140	138	mmol/L
(137-147)					
Potass.	4.4	4.4	4.4	4.3	mmol/L
(3.5-5.0)					
Chloride	105	102	104	103	mmol/L
(96-109)					
Bicarb	27	29	27	28	mmol/L
(25-33)					
An.Gap	16	11	13	11	mmol/L
(4-17)					
Gluc	6.1	5.7	5.5	5.6	mmol/L
(3.0-6.0)					
Urea	5.7	6.3	5.0	5.1	mmol/L
(3.0-8.5)					
Creat	69	82	68	69	umol/L
(60-140)					
eGFR	> 90	> 90	> 90	> 90	mL/min (over
59)					
Urate	0.39	0.43	0.45	0.39	mmol/L
(0.12-0.45)					
T.Bili	5	9	9	8	umol/L
(2-20)					
Alk.P	57	51	43	48	U/L
(30-115)					

If you suffer from Depression, and are sceptical about my advice on salt, go and get an ION test to see what your salt levels are.

If they're at the bottom of the range, or lower, then I suggest you try my salt experiment.

Salt, as stated before, is how electrical signals move throughout your body. The less salt you have in your system, the slower the signals move. Slow signals can result in Depression and anxiety.

Now there's a slight problem with lab tests on salt. It has nothing to do with the tests themselves, but your body has an inbuilt ability to hang on to salt/ to conserve it. Unless you're an athlete, very unwell, or you drink crazy amounts of water quickly, your body will cling onto the salt for dear life. It's unlikely that your body will fall out of the ranges for salt (on the downside). In short, the lab tests will rarely show Hyponatremia. All the studies show that given free availability of salt, almost everyone will fall into the range of 6-12g of salt per day, with the sweet spot being around 10g per day for an adult. That's the place where your body runs at optimum levels, and that is what I believe you should aim for. Give it a try for a few weeks and see how you go. If you don't feel that it's doing you any good, then go back to where you were before.

Japan and Switzerland

The two countries with the longest life expectancy are Japan and Switzerland.

The two countries with the highest per capita incomes are Japan and Switzerland.

The two fully-developed countries with the highest salt consumption are Japan and Switzerland.

The part of the world with the lowest salt consumption is Central Africa.

The part of the world with the lowest life expectancy is Central Africa.

The part of the world with the lowest per capita income is Central Africa.

Here's something I just discovered. It's claimed by various authorities like WHO (World Health Organisation) and the American Heart Foundation that salt is bad for you, because it leads to hypertension (high blood pressure) and cardiovascular disease. However, if you look at a reliable source like *Worldlifeexpectancy.com*, you'll find that deaths from Cardiovascular disease or hypertension are low in both Japan and Switzerland. Japan ranks 182/183 for coronary heart disease deaths, and Switzerland ranks 167/183.

Japan is 183/183 for hypertension deaths, and Switzerland is 125/183.

This shouldn't be directly translated as a hard rule, but when you see statistics like this, you should pay attention.

Now I also did a bit of research on the major civilisations around the world, over the last few thousand years. I'm not going to get into the specifics here because in terms of Depression, it's not that important. What I did find though, was the importance of salt, and the salt trade to all of those cultures. From what I can make out, the best quality salts are mined from ancient, dried-up oceans or seas that have then been folded under pressure by movements in the earth's crust. This causes the salt crystals to take on the colour and benefits of other minerals contained within the salt crystal, particularly Potassium and Iodine.

I don't have much information about the salt and Depression link, but there are studies to show salt as the best thing to lower Cortisol. Cortisol, we will discuss later, but it's basically your stress hormone. More Cortisol = More Stress.

Salt is a 'Natural Mood-booster'

Scientists suggest that we may add extra salt to our food because it boosts our mood, even though we have been taught that too much is bad for us. The University of Iowa researchers writing in Psychology and Behaviour say salt may act as a natural antidepressant. Tests on rats found those with a salt deficiency shied away from activities they normally enjoyed – a sign of Depression.

The University of Haifa studied students and found particularly in women, that adding salt to their food may have anti-depressant effects. Salt slows down the destruction of serotonin and dopamine. The reason women are most prone to adding salt is because they tend to consume less salt in their diets, compared to men. This is likely due to low salt guidelines recommended by health authorities. Women are good at following dietary recommendations, men aren't.

Graph 3 (below): Again, this graph shows the sweet spot for salt is around 11gms per day. It's interesting to note that by exceeding this amount, shows only a small risk of premature death, whereas reducing the salt intake quickly places you into risky territory. In other words... higher amount of salt; not so bad...lower amount of salt; not good.

GRAPH 3.

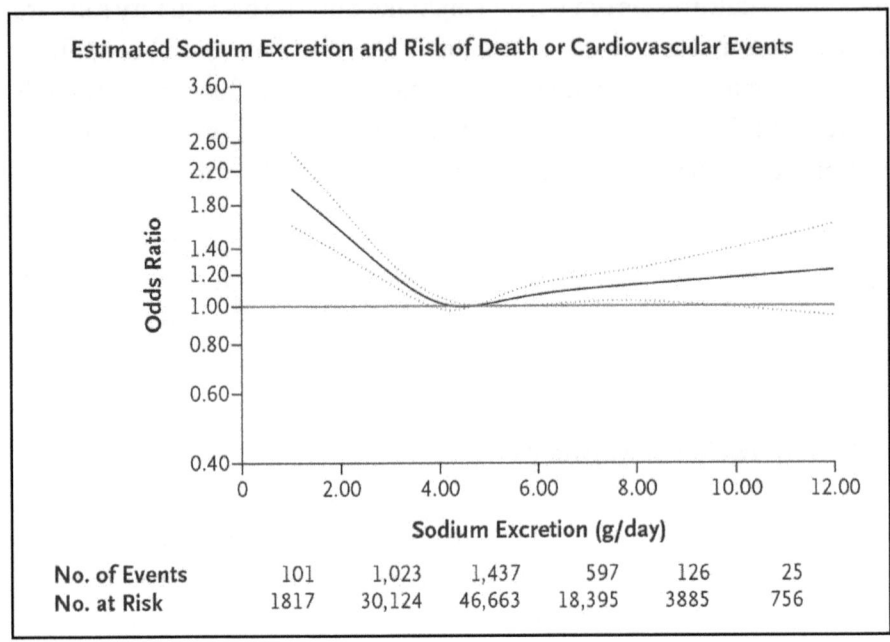

(Web source: https://www.nejm.org/doi/full/10.1056/NEJMoa1311889)

It's almost impossible to meet the recommended low sodium guidelines of 1500mg per day, up to 2300mg maximum. That's only about ½ to 1 teaspoon of salt per day.

Salt is absolutely essential to life and your body contains about 250g of it. You use up salt daily as you sweat and you must replace it from external sources. Your body cannot make it. The current hysteria surrounding salt, in my opinion, is quite wrong. Salt was prized in the ancient world, even traded as a type of currency. Salzburg, a lovely town in Austria, literally means 'salt fortress/salt city' and became the 'Fort Knox' of

Rome. I mean don't overdo it with salt, but it's certainly not the enemy. If you want to start feeling depressed, eat a bland diet with low salt and I'm pretty sure you'll start feeling unhappy. Food is supposed to taste good, and we all know that good tasting food makes us happy. Salt away, but don't overdo it, and go for a quality type.

The 'Good' Bermuda Triangle of Salt (Vienna)

Salzburg, as mentioned above, is an awesome city. I've been there a few times. I haven't seen one part of Austria that I don't like (yet). If this country was in Queensland, I'd live in it, but I digress. Salzburg was a fortified city built by the Romans to protect their salt. Those Romans must have been pretty dumb to build a fortress city around salt. I mean you'd think it was gold. Oh, I forgot, you can't eat gold, but you can eat salt.

Here's two Romans, sitting having a beer after work:

> "What's your job mate?"
> "Oh, I'm a guard at the bank vault. I protect the gold bullion."
> "Is that all? I'm a guard at the salt supply, now that's a serious job."

Yep, those Romans built a walled city to protect salt, while the crooks were taking off with the gold! There were times in history when gold and salt were by weight, interchangeable. That is, salt was worth the same as gold.

The word 'salary' derives from the Latin word 'sal'. You guessed it … sal is the Latin word for salt. I guess we'll employ that guy for a week and see if he's 'worth his salt'. If it works out, we'll pay him a good salary, if it doesn't, we feel that his work is hardly worth 'a grain of salt'. Or maybe he's 'the salt of the earth' or just a 'good old salt'. Here's another good one … a word for healthy or wholesome in Latin is 'salus', which come from the word 'sal' (SALT).

It just seems to me that perhaps this salt stuff is pretty important.

My theory is that many depressed people have a chronically low level of salt. Hey, go to the doctor and take the test, it's not hard.

I've been banging on about the importance of salt in Austria/Southern Germany, the Romans' salt supply city. So here's something else to think about. Who has been the smartest guy to inhabit the earth in say the last hundred years? The answer would probably be, and should be, Albert Einstein.

Einstein was born in Germany and moved to Munich when he was a year old. From here he moved to Switzerland during his early years, then back to Berlin, before eventually settling in the USA (because of the war/being a Jew, etc). Now if you look at other famous/influential people from Salzburg, Munich, the Vienna Triangle, and the Bermuda Triangle of Europe, these are some of the names you'll find.

Mozart, Hitler, Schwarzenegger (maybe not an intellectual genius, but pretty accomplished), Strauss, and Beethoven. Beethoven was born in central Germany, but moved to Vienna, Austria at age 21. Archduke Ferdinand from Vienna, allegedly caused the First World War. Sigmund Freud, Carl Jung (psychiatrist), Marie Antionette, Nietzsche (philosopher), Wagner (composer), Humboldt (who basically invented school as we know it, amongst many other things), Gutenberg (inventor of the printing press), and Martin Luther (who started non-Catholic Christianity. I'm not saying they're all good people, but they are powerful and influential. Each has contributed in shaping the fantastic world that we enjoy today. Don't get me wrong, there are plenty of cities where 'smart' people are brought together. London is a magnet for them, so too is Silicon Valley. Still, there's something very important about salt, and if you look into the history of it, you'll find out even more. That being said, if you can find a group of more talented, influential or enlightened individuals, all born in such close proximity within the last 500 years, you'll be doing well.

Rome was another centre of major achievement. Their salt was carried from Austria, along Roman-built roads known as the 'Salt Roads', designed primarily for the transportation of salt.

Apart from influential people, have a look at the companies who are headquartered, or originated from the areas surrounding Salzburg and Munich: BMW, Mercedes Benz, Porsche, Bayer (chemicals and pharmaceuticals), Allianz (the world's largest insurance company), and one of my personal favourites; Hirmer. They're the world's largest menswear store. Red Bull (the drink) also has its headquarters in Salzburg. Siemens, Europe's largest manufacturer of instrumentation and control systems, also has its headquarters in Munich. If you go to the Deutsches Museum in Munich, you'll see that the Germans invented everything except paper (that was the Egyptians). But, the Germans did improve paper quality, so it became very useful. In turn, they followed up with the invention of the first printing press (Gutenburg).

On a recent visit to Austria, I visited some of the salt mines. The original workers mined salt from hundreds of metres below the surface, for thousands of years. The conditions would have been very difficult. People wouldn't go underground and risk their lives for salt, unless it was important. Those that controlled the salt trade were the wealthiest people in the land.

Here's another anecdotal study I found.

The Astronaut Urine Study
(Web source: https://www.ncbi.nlm.nih.gov/pmc/articles/PMC5409798/)

Performed on men who were in training for space missions. They basically lived in a self-sufficient bubble and were studied to see how they reacted to their conditions.

One of the researchers was looking at Urine volumes, as you do.

He found that the astronauts with the highest salt intake had the greatest urine volumes, regardless of their fluid intake. It remained the same as the other men. The astronauts with the higher salt intake actually reported being less thirsty than the lower salt intake astronauts. So realistically, if you drink say two litres of fluid, then you should wee out around 1.8 litres. The remainder is either breathed out or perspired (don't quote me on numbers). But the astronauts with higher salt intakes weed out more like 2.2 litres and still exhaled moisture and perspired. The water had to come from somewhere. The theory is that when the salt content rises (outside the cell), the cell then fights to maintain the same saltiness inside the cell. It does this by forcing water out of the cell and into the body (it's called osmotic pressure). It's then excreted in the form of urine.

Let's say it this way; the formerly bloated cell starts losing water inside the cell, then disposes of the excess water. Therefore, the astronauts should also lose weight. The weird thing… it was also found in similar animal models, that the animals with the higher salt content could eat 25% more calories and still maintain the same body weight. In my language that means the higher salt content increased the animals' rate of metabolism.

Now this isn't relevant to Depression per se, but there may be some clues here in relation to salt consumption and obesity.

As I said in an earlier chapter, do the experiment. Up your salt intake a bit and see what happens. Maybe your weight goes down, and maybe your Depression reduces. Do your own research if you like, but salt matters.

Magnesium Salt

Experts suggest that we're all low in Magnesium these days, so many people take magnesium supplements and magnesium baths. I don't know if we're all low in magnesium or not, but it may well be the case. The point I would like to make is that sodium and chloride are more important and easier to obtain. So, if you take a magnesium supplement for a week, or a month, you most likely have enough magnesium for a while. Perhaps you take a little bit every now and then. Again, I don't know the answer. The magnesium usually comes in salt form, like Epsom Salts (also called magnesium sulphate). My personal view is that the sulphur is more important than the magnesium, but I digress again. When you take a standard blood test, you're not commonly tested for magnesium. Perhaps it's because it just isn't that important, again I don't know…it's just a suggestion. Do you know what's important? Your salt level - sodium and chloride, and it's such an easy thing to fix too. It's also easy to be diverted away from the fundamentals, and latch on to the next big thing. I've been caught in those traps myself; you know chugging down superfoods and upping doses of magnesium. There may well be something in it, but don't forget the salt.

Lithium Salt

Lithium's a rare metal and your body likes a little of it, but not too much. Lithium was one of the first antidepressants used, and is still used today. It's possible to purchase lithium supplements over the counter. Lithium appears to regulate neurotransmitters such as GABA and Dopamine. So, following are a couple of fun facts regarding lithium.

The soda drink '7Up' used to contain lithium until about 1950. Seven (7) is the atomic number of lithium. For those unfamiliar with chemistry, lithium is the seventh heaviest element. Hydrogen is the lightest; atomic number 1. The 'Up' refers to the 'lift' you get from drinking 7Up.

In Europe and America for centuries it was common to visit natural spas. They were said to be good for your health. Many of the spa waters were high in lithium, which allegedly makes you feel good. One example is Lithia Springs in Georgia, USA. Lithia Springs seems to have been a sacred site for native American Indians.

Two studies were undertaken; one in Texas and one in Japan. The counties or provinces with the highest, natural lithium content in their water, correlated exactly with the lowest death rates from Depression, and the lowest levels of violent crime.

(Web Source: https://www.ncbi.nlm.nih.gov/pmc/articles/PMC3863886/)

There have been other studies and they mostly seem to draw the same conclusion. That's not to say that there isn't room for scepticism, just that it seems to come up over and over again.

What I say is give some lithium salt a try, just don't overdo it.

Coincidentally , Lithium was the first ever anti-depressant drug, and it's still being used today.

Iodine

Iodine is strongly related to your thyroid gland, which is like the master metaboliser. If your thyroid is not functioning well (which is common enough), then you may not be producing neurotransmitters properly, so in turn, not getting the best out of your food supply. Iodine is so important that almost all advanced countries add iodine routinely to their salt supply. A hundred years ago, iodine deficiency was extremely common, especially in areas where farming was conducted in low iodine soils. This included large parts of the southern USA, Asia, New Zealand, and Australia (especially Tasmania). In fact, adding Iodine to the salt supply appeared to increase the IQ of children by about 15 points, which is huge. From what I can make out, Iodine deficiency is probably the world's most prevalent mineral deficiency, with possibly two billion people affected. Iodised salt is much less popular today, but that doesn't mean that Iodine is less important than it was back then. Getting plenty of iodine is definitely a worthwhile exercise.

The easiest way to get some iodine is to eat iodised salt. It may not be enough, but it's a start.

The thing is, in this book we're not dealing with general health, but with Depression. Firstly on that issue, I would say, as I have throughout this book, that general health and mental health are inextricably linked (cannot be separated). Secondly, there are some strong studies linking salt/s and mood.

SPOOKY STORIES

- SALT IN INDIA -

Salt was the reason Britain lost India. That's an exaggeration, but not by much.

The English banned the Indians from harvesting their own salt, which they'd done for thousands of years. They wanted to sell the Indians salt imported from England, which was highly taxed. Salt taxes provided almost 10% of the Government budget in India.

Ghandi led a march across India and when he reached the coast, he ceremoniously harvested salt, which was illegal at the time. Ghandi had cleverly chosen salt as the focus of his protest movement because salt was something that affected everyone, rich and poor, hindu and muslim, alike.

Explaining his choice to use salt as the focus, Gandhi said, *"Next to air and water, salt is perhaps the greatest necessity of life."*

- SALT RULES! -

In my serum Biochemistry results a few pages back, have a look at the actual numbers. For example, sodium should be about 140mmol/l, Potassium is 4mmol/litre. Chloride is 100mmol/litre, Bicarbonate is 30mmol/litre. These numbers are not simply comparable, but close enough. So the sodium is 140mmol/l, the chloride is 100mmol/l and the next most important is potassium at 4mmol/l. Okay, bicarbonate is also important at 30mmol/l, but the salt is where the action is.

Salt is 250 mmol/l, and magnesium sulphate would be 10mmol/litre (or thereabouts). In other words I would say this...lithium, magnesium, iodine, and potassium are all important, but make sure you get enough salt.

CHAPTER 12

Vitamins

Vitamins, and vitamin supplements can be tricky. It's not just because the quality varies so much, it is also a matter of how your body responds to them, and I'm not talking about you as an individual, or your genetics. So how does your body deal with a concentrated form of vitamin that was only previously found in a food?

Generally speaking, very little of a vitamin tablet contains actual vitamin. The overwhelming majority of the tablet is made up of fillers. Take vitamin B12 for example: a fairly high dose is 500mcg, or 500 divided by 1000 divided by 1000 grams. 1g is pretty small. Imagine your tablet weighs around half a gram. That means the vitamin content isn't even 1% of that tablet, it's more like 0.1%. So 99.9% of your tablet is something else, other than B12, fillers in other words. That varies depending on the vitamin, but except in the case of vitamin C, not by too much.

Here's a little joke about that - it applies to food. Check the sugar content of your tomato sauce. It's usually 25% sugar. Peanut butter is usually around 10% sugar. Most Asian sauces and BBQ sauces are higher again, like 40 or 50%. Sweet chilli sauce is my favourite, but it should be called 'sugar sauce with chilli flavouring', because it is 60%+ sugar. In the case of vitamin B tablets, there isn't enough vitamin B to even give it a vitamin B flavour. The tablet is basically 99% rice starch or magnesium stearate, or some other allegedly inert chemical.

Let's look at something simple to begin with, like vitamin C. An orange contains 75mg of vitamin C, but an orange also contains fibre, flavonoids, water, minerals, etc. When you take a 1000mg vitamin C tablet, it's the equivalent of 14 oranges in terms of vitamin C, but has none of the other components that an orange has. How does your body deal with this? The answer is that we just don't know. All we do know is that we piss most of it out. It's still putting an unnecessary load on the body.

Here's another good one; vitamin A. It's a fat-soluble vitamin, so unlike Vitamin C, we can't just piss it out. Vitamin A is great for your eyesight. The reason there's an epidemic of blindness in South East Asia is a lack of vitamin A amongst the poorest people. Vitamin A is mainly found in meat, fish, and animal fat. These foods are the most expensive component of their diets, so the poor just don't eat them, and blindness can follow thereafter. On the other hand, excess vitamin A will kill you. The explorers who accompanied Mawson, racing to be the first to the South Pole, died on the homeward trip. They were starving and ate their dogs' livers, which contain huge amounts of vitamin A. The explorers died of vitamin A poisoning, which is horrific apparently. The point being, vitamins can help and heal, but also kill you. When you take a concentrated form of any vitamin, you have no idea what is going to happen. You won't die from it, but does your body really need it? And is it causing stress to your body?

If you take something that works for you, then by all means keep taking it. What I want to talk about is the huge variability in supplement quality (not just based on price) and how choosing the wrong supplement may be affecting your mental health.

Vitamin B

Vitamin B is 'seemingly' about eight different vitamins rolled into one:

B1   Thiamine
B2   Riboflavin
B3   Niacin
B5   Pantothenic Acid
B6   Pyridoxine
B7   Biotin
B9   Folate
B12 Cobalamin

Most people have heard of Folic acid; it's known as vitamin B9 (and sometimes as Folate), but it isn't. Folic acid is a synthetic substance that didn't exist until seventy years ago. Folic acid has a similar, though not identical chemical formula to Folate (real natural B9). Some Folic acid is converted into Folate in the body. But some people (around 40% of the population) have a 'gene mutation' that prevents this conversion of Folic acid to Folate. What's worse is that undigested Folic acid circulates in the system and builds up. Undigested Folic acid also prevents the uptake of real Folate. There is substantial evidence that undigested Folic acid causes some cancers and the prevalence is statistically significant, like a 25% higher chance of particular cancers. 'Natural' Folate can now be made into a tablet, but this technology is only about fifteen years old.

So why doesn't all B9 come in 'natural' form? Well, for the most part, it's about the price. Even if you don't take Folic acid in a vitamin or multivitamin, you're being force-fed it. Folic acid is added to all commercial flours (bread, muffins, pasta, pizza bases, bagels) in the USA, Australia, New Zealand, Canada, and the UK, at least. Folic acid is best known for its ability to prevent neural tube defects in babies, so women are advised to take B9 during pregnancy. That seems like a good thing, so there are benefits.

People with the 'gene defect' have actually been found to show great alleviation from Depression (especially anxiety) when they avoid Folic acid and substitute it with 'natural Folate' (also known as 5-MTHF, or Methyl Tetra Hyrdra Folate). The best thing you can do is to get your

Folate from natural foods like leafy greens, or beef liver, if you can stand it. I know that I have the 'gene defect' because I've been tested. This test is free in Australia.

Now we could go into all kinds of medical or natural 'cures' for these problems, but the best thing to do, as I've said, is get your Folate from real food. The other takeaway is that vitamin supplements can both heal and harm.

I've read about a few people who've overcome their anxiety quickly, just by changing over to 5-MTHF (natural folate). You can look up a great article here:

(Web source: https://www.adelaidenow.com.au/lifestyle/sa-weekend/how-a-vitamin-cured-my-anxiety-elisa-blacks-story-of-lifelong-struggle-and-new-hope-for-the-future/news-story/058666cc 978da7ee1fca0f1ee043212c)

Vitamin B12

Like B9, many similar problems arise in relation to B12. The vitamin B12 commonly sold in supplements is Cyanocobalamin. This is a synthetic molecule that didn't exist until seventy years ago. Chemically, it's similar to 'real' vitamin B12, but not the same. 'Real' vitamin B12 is Methylcobalamin, and it can be purchased at a pharmacy, but only occurs in around 5% of the formulas.

I know that Cyanocobalamin (synthetic vitamin B12) personally causes a rapid mood drop for me, like within an hour. My children, who have also inherited my 'gene defect' notice it too. You'll notice that I've placed 'gene defect' in inverted commas, because I don't look upon it as a 'defect' at all. About 40% of the population has this 'defect'. It means that we have trouble metabolising synthetic B vitamin products that didn't exist seventy years ago, so not much of a defect really. It's like putting diesel fuel into a petrol car, thinking it will work just as well.

Other B Vitamins

All the other B vitamins come in either an 'active' or 'passive' form. Unless you're taking a high end expensive product, you'll generally only be receiving the 'passive' form. That may be good for you, but it may not be. I don't have all the answers. If you feel something that has been recommended to you works, then keep doing it. If you have Depression or anxiety however, there's a possibility that it could stem partly from a vitamin or substance that you're ingesting, intentionally or not.

When I was a boy, it seemed like technology would deliver us all sorts of benefits including nutritional ones. Instead of mucking about with eating and cooking, we'd just be able to take a tablet with all the nutrients we needed, then we could have much more time to play footy, watch TV, surf, and even chase girls. Well it didn't work out that way. It seems that the more we learned about nutrition and attempted to 'science our way' out of cooking and eating, the further we strayed from real nutrition.

And another thing... if you stand outside a vitamin C factory for example, you'll hardly see trucks carrying oranges and lemons lined up to offload their cargo. Most vitamin C is made from petrochemicals and other industrial compounds. Vitamin B9 (folate) is not made from spinach. Vitamin A is not made from carrots or beef liver. Vitamin D is not made from sunshine or cod livers. In regard to all vitamin supplements, you need to be a bit more careful and discerning. Sometimes it doesn't matter, but often it does.

Vitamin C

An average orange contains 75mg of vitamin C. A typical vitamin C tablet contains 500 to 1000mg of vitamin C. A very respected vitamin company in Australia makes a 1000mg tablet and recommends one per day, or three per day if a cold is coming on. So the daily dose is 14 oranges, or 42 oranges if you have a sniffle. I'd suggest that if you consumed 42 oranges, you wouldn't have to be worried about a cold, you'd be much sicker from the oranges. If you need 42 oranges to ward off a cold, perhaps their vitamin C isn't as potent as it should be. Does eating the equivalent of 42 oranges without the balancing effect of fibre and sugars, cause other bodily problems? I don't know the answer. There are plenty of studies showing high doses of vitamin C work for a cold, but maybe just eating two oranges would be better and easier on your body. Again, I'm not sure, but I'm thinking about it.

Vitamins from Animal Products

Pound for pound, or gram for gram, animal products are the top food source of every vitamin, except for vitamin C. All the sources of vitamins from animals are in their natural form, and the most absorbable.

Liver compared to Fruit and Vegetables

	Apple (100 g)	Carrots (100g)	Red Meat (100g)	Beef Liver (100g)
Calcium	3.0 mg	3.3 mg	11.0 mg	11.0 mg
Phosphorus	6.0 mg	31.0 mg	140.0 mg	476.0 mg
Magnesium	4.8 mg	6.2 mg	15.0 mg	18.0 mg
Potassium	139.0 mg	222.0 mg	370.0 mg	380.0 mg
Iron	.1 mg	.6 mg	3.3 mg	8.8 mg
Zinc	.05 mg	.3 mg	4.4 mg	4.0 mg
Copper	.04 mg	.08 mg	.18 mg	12.0 mg
Vitamin A	None	None	40 IU	53,400 IU
Vitamin D	None	None	Trace	19 IU
Vitamin E	.37 mg	.11 mg	1.7 mg	.63 mg
Vitamin C	7.0 mg	6.0 mg	None	27.0 mg
Thiamin	.03 mg	.05 mg	.05 mg	.26 mg
Riboflavin	.02 mg	.05 mg	.20 mg	4.19 mg
Niacin	.10 mg	.60 mg	4.0 mg	16.5 mg
Pantothenic Acid	.11 mg	.19 mg	.42 mg	8.8 mg

	Apple (100 g)	Carrots (100g)	Red Meat (100g)	Beef Liver (100g)
Vitamin B6	.03 mg	.10 mg	.07 mg	.73 mg
Folate	8.0 mcg	24.0 mcg	4.0 mcg	145.0 mcg
Biotin	None	.42 mcg	2.08 mcg	96.0 mcg
Vitamin B12	None	None	1.84 mcg	111.3 mcg

(Web source: https://chriskresser.com/natures-most-potent-superfood/)

A word on liver supplements...if you really want a vitamin tablet that works, go for dessicated liver from grass-fed animals (or real liver if you have the guts).

Vitamin tablets are okay and occasionally they're helpful. I wouldn't take them every day though. Also check to see if they are naturally derived, or some other synthetic chemical. Be aware of the concentration too; 'more' doesn't necessarily mean 'better'. Obtain your vitamins from food whenever possible.

SPOOKY STORIES

- VITAMINS -

Gut bacteria will make vitamins for you.

Almost all B vitamins can be made by gut bacteria, as can vitamin K.

Fermenting cabbage appears to increase the vitamin C content of the cabbage by up to 30x the original cabbage. When Captain Cook sailed the world, he first discovered limes as a source of vitamin C to prevent Scurvy. He didn't know it was vitamin C at the time, it hadn't been discovered yet. Limes were not easy to come by, but sauerkraut was. Sauerkraut replaced limes and that worked too.

CHAPTER 13

Vegans + Vegetarians

I doubt that any vegans or vegetarians have made it to this point in the book...almost everything I've said about Depression and diet, is aimed against these guys. BUT...I had an epiphany yesterday about how these guys survive. I say this because on paper, there's no reason they should survive long term, and no historical/anthropological evidence of a vegan diet ever working.

I mean, I'm not saying it can't be done, obviously it can. It's just that without our modern availability of food, calories, and possibly supplements, it would be totally unsustainable. Meat-eaters would just outcompete vegetarians every time, on a species-wide scale. That doesn't mean that vegetarians can't be better runners, swimmers or tennis players...they can be. But when left to nature's ravages, vegetarians and vegans would be outbred by the meat-eaters within a generation or two. Fortunately, the modern world has provided great bounty, so that vegetarians and vegans can survive (as crazy as that concept is). Here's an example of vegetarians in nature: Some animals that are vegetarians; cows, monkeys, and rabbits. Here are a few animals that are carnivores; dogs, cats, lions, tigers, wolves, and dolphins.

So, given the opportunity to be reincarnated, would you choose to be a lion or a rabbit? Anyway, I'll leave you to ponder that on your own... but I choose a lion, or a dolphin.

Vegan Cats

There's a great story by Joe Rogan (a comedian/health blogger) about vegan cats. I don't know if it's true, but I suspect it is. The story goes like this: Some vegans keep cats as pets, and many of these vegans (people) also feed their cats a vegan diet. According to Joe, these cats live for a long and healthy four years. Now regular cats have an average lifespan of fifteen years. The difference is the physical and chemical structure of their digestive systems. It's also largely influenced by the bacteria in the cat's gut. A cat's gut is very similar in construction to a human gut. The point is that cats are meant be carnivores, not vegans. Cats can live on a vegan diet, but not for very long. Humans are omnivores, and much closer to being carnivores than being vegetarians. Humans' guts are also far closer to that of a dog, another (mostly) carnivore, than say to a monkey, a rabbit or a cow.

I know it's all a bit harsh, but here's the real point of the issue. The reason that humans built the colosseum, created language, religion, cities and societies, is because they eat meat, and they cook it. Monkeys are still hanging out in the trees because they spend all day (like 18 hours) chewing and gathering food. It's that simple! Humans were relieved of this problem thousands of years ago because they ate calorie-dense food (meat) and unlocked the potential of the food by cooking it. Cooking predigests the food, thereby making it easier to extract the calories. Humans are the only animals that have learned to cook. You should eat what you have evolved to eat, basically a mixture of cooked and raw meat, and vegetables when you have to.

Indian Dilemma

Now I've struggled for a long time with the Indian dilemma. Having been to India, and discovered that many of them are vegetarian or vegan, AND, that they've been around forever, AND, there are so many of them, it just didn't make sense. So here's the rub. Until last century, Indian people ate animals, except the cow of course, but they did eat everything that came out of the cow. The cow is sacred, not from anything that God told them, but because everything that comes from the cow is so precious, like milk, butter, oil, cheese and calories. The cow is revered because its products are so life giving and healthful. Since many Indians have become fully vegan, their health problems are rising off the charts. Obesity, diabetes, and cancer, are significantly increasing now that they've stopped using animal products to sustain themselves. In particular, they've replaced dairy based cooking oil (Ghee, butter) with much cheaper, so-called vegetable oils.

Vegetarians and Cancer

Now let's take a look at a study from England. 30,000 vegetarians were followed for a few years and compared to 30,000 non-vegetarians. The study found that cancer rates were lower by about 11% in the vegetarians (score one for the veggos!). This makes perfect sense because the non-vegetarians are probably not that 'health conscious'. They also probably drink more, smoke more, and exercise less. They likely eat more take away food too. 11% is not a huge difference, but it's better than zero. What the study also found was that Bowel Cancer was 40% higher in the vegetarian group! 40%! Now that's a big number. This number is telling us that vegetarianism is not the natural order of things. The vegetables upset the gut and are not easily processed. This is the opposite of what we've been told. We're told that meat is the cause of colon/bowel cancer. The study states that this information is incorrect. Just indulge me (again) for a minute … I like numbers, but not everyone does. Let's assume that of the two groups above (there were 30,000 vegetarians and 30,000 non-vegetarians), the overall cancer rate during the study was say 30/100 (or thirty out of one hundred), in the vegetarian group. The non-veg group was then about 33/100: different, but not by much. When it comes to bowel cancer only, the non-veg group was say 20/100, and the veg group was almost 30/100 (actually 28/100). That's a huge and significant difference.

(Web source: https://www.ncbi.nlm.nih.gov/pmc/articles/PMC2699384/)

Now I, along with the study, aren't suggesting you don't eat vegetables. Vegetables are great and very healthy. What I believe the study is telling us: DON'T ONLY EAT VEGETABLES, all the time. Again, it may seem harsh but your body loves meat. Most meat will contain at least double the calories of any plant food by weight. For example: 100gms of beef = 250 calories, 100gms of mango = 60 calories.

Here's the epiphany I mentioned that I had yesterday. It was that vegans and vegetarians survive (and thrive) because of the animals they eat. WHAT? Yep, it's the bacteria in their guts. As you now know, bacteria are sort of like tiny animals and they're full of protein and vitamins. The bacteria inside a vegan's colon struggle (which is why their bowel cancer rates are higher), but bacteria are so adaptable, they just do what they have to, to help their host survive. Like I say, it's not the natural order of things, but these bacteria babies do the best they can with what they're given.

Calorie Density

Until very recently in human history, obtaining sufficient calories was the primary aim of most people. So, with the resources they had available, along with the time it took to harness those resources, humans required as many calories as they could get, in the most efficient way. That basically meant minimising the amount of time it took to stuff calories into their mouths. Again, may seem harsh, but our ancestors were doing this for thousands of years before we came along. You'd better get used to it. Your body much prefers dense calories over weak ones. Your body loves meat.

I Didn't Make The Rules

I developed a challenge in my mind while writing this book. It's like a reality TV show (not *Survivor*). Let's call it 'Survival' or maybe 'The Last Supper' (take your pick). The loser starves or dies, so it's not quite as much fun as the TV versions.

It goes something like this: Three competitors ... I place a table in front of them with three foods on it. One's a bowl of raw, untrimmed steak, another is a bowl of fruit and vegetables, and the third is a bowl of wheat. Each competitor can choose only one bowl. They then have to walk to the next destination, three days away, where the same food will be offered. Just to show that I'm humane, I allow them an hour to cook and eat, and have sufficient water to take with them.

Let's assume for arguments sake that each meal contains the same number of calories (let's say 3000 calories). Which bowl should they choose? Well it wouldn't be the wheat, because that's basically poison and will make them sick. The only reason that we can eat wheat is due to the milling of it, turning that into bread by fermentation. The same goes for almost any grain. Grains must be pre-digested in some way for us to gain nutrition from them.

Anyway, they could choose either the meat, or the veggies, and they'd probably make it to the next destination. Once there, they're presented with the same choices, three days later. Again, they cook and eat their chosen food then set off back to the first table. They trek back and forth until there's only one person left. I'll tell you who wins this game ... it's the competitor who eats the meat. Strangely enough, this game has been played for centuries. We ate meat when we could get it. When we couldn't, we ate vegetables. If we couldn't get them either, we'd eat grass or grain, or dirt if we had to. Keep in mind that in the 'real life' game, we had to compete as well, and when times got tough, there was plenty of competition.

Vegetable Oil

There's no such thing as vegetable oil. Have a look at your bottle. What is the oil made from? My bet is ... not a vegetable. Vegetables are things like zucchini, broccoli, carrots, spinach, collard greens, eggplant, beans (not really, but close). I'm guessing your vegetable oil is made from coconuts, soy, canola, peanuts, sunflower, safflower, rice bran, and whatever else. None of these things are vegetables, or even resemble them. Just in case I'm asked, and I will be, olives are not vegetables. Olives are a fruit, so olive oil, which is about the healthiest of all non-animal oils, is a fruit oil. Avocado and macadamia are good oils too, but neither of them are vegetables.

All so-called vegetable oils, I class as poisons. They're made from plants that either didn't exist fifty years ago (Canola for example), or certainly weren't in abundance (soy), and rely on modern farming methods and powerful industrial processes for their existence (sunflower, rice bran).

Generally vegetable oils are mostly Omega 6 oils. Omega 6, 3, and other oils looks like this.

Possibly, you've been sold the idea that poly-unsaturated oils are the way to go. It even sounds healthy. What poly-unsaturated means is that there are 'multiple sites' (poly) where the double bond is present. Mono-unsaturated fats like macadamia and avocado oils, are considered very healthy, but they're expensive too. The 'mono' means only one double bond carbon to carbon. In contrast, 'poly' means multiple double bonds. Double bonds are unstable and easily oxidised by heat. Believe me, this is bad. The reason you can only use vegetable oil once or twice, is that heating it tends to oxidise it, which sort of destroys the oil, making it unhealthy.

The more poly-unsaturated the oil, the more unstable it is. All vegetable oils are mostly poly-unsaturated.

The only oils that are really considered stable at temperature are saturated oils. They can be used again and again if temperatures are maintained at around 200 degrees. Saturated sounds awful, fatty, or gluey, but it doesn't mean that at all. 'Saturated' just means that the oil is saturated with strong hydrogen bonds and won't oxidise easily.

Many people will say, "I just avoid fats and oils and try to cook without it, to limit my oil intake." Bzzzzz...wrong answer. Oil is absolutely essential to life. All of your cell walls and even your brain is made from oil/fat/cholesterol.

Why is this important if you have Depression? Because your brain health is reliant on saturated fat and cholesterol, and the right balance of Omega 6 and Omega 3 oils. But, the omega 3 oils found in vegetables are not the kind of Omega 3 oils that your brain needs.

The three main omega-3 fatty acids are: alpha-linolenic acid (ALA), eicosapentaenoic acid (EPA), and docosahexaenoic acid (DHA). ALA is the type of Omega 3 found in plants (mostly). Your brain is not made from ALA, it's made from EPA and DHA. This is the type of Omega 3 contained in fish oil tablets, you know, the ones that enhance your brain health and cognitive function. They do work, but you have to limit Omega 6, otherwise the flood of it overwhelms the trickle of Omega 3.

EPA and DHA are the type of Omega 3 found in cod liver oil and all of the prized foods like caviar, tuna, salmon, fatty beef, eggs, raw cheeses, anchovies, sardines, oysters, and lobsters.

It's virtually impossible to get DHA and EPA from vegetarian sources, except for some algae. Even then you'd need modern processing methods to refine it. Omega 3 from algae was only discovered a few short years ago.

Vegetables and Vitamins

With the exception of vitamin C (which is a special case), you'll find that the top sources of each vitamin are meat, or animal sources.

So, for example, the top sources of vitamin B12 will be cow's liver, followed by beef, fish, oysters, lamb pork, etc. It's the same for every vitamin and most minerals too. The word Folate (B9) comes from the Latin word 'folium', which means leaf. The largest source of this vitamin though, is still meat, and animal products.

'Popeye' ate spinach for the energy it gave him, supposedly from the iron and folate. He would have been far better off to have a small serving of calves' liver.

An article from *Medical News Today*:

> *"Recommended Intake of Vitamin A. There are two main types of vitamin A:*
>
> *Preformed vitamin A: This comes in the form of retinol and is present in animal-based food sources, including meat, fish, poultry, and dairy products.*
>
> *Provitamin A: This comes in the form of carotenoids, mainly beta carotene. It is present in plant-based foods, such as fruits and vegetables.*
>
> *To aid the absorption of vitamin A, a person needs to include some fat in their diet. It is also important not to overcook foods, as this reduces the vitamin A contents."*

I also found this list in *Medical News Today*:

Assume the amounts are based on an average serve. So with meat it's 3ozs (100grams) and for vegetables, it's about a cup.

"The Top Sources of Vitamin A:

Beef liver	*6500mcg*
Cod liver oil - 1 tspn	*4000mcg*
Sweet potato	*1400mcg*
Carrots	*460mcg*
Broccoli	*120mcg*
Mango	*110mcg."*

(Web source: https://www.medicalnewstoday.com/articles/219486)

In other words, beef liver contains sixty times the vitamin A found in mangoes, and fifteen times that of carrots. Even if you ate the carrots, you're not getting 'real' vitamin A, and the conversion rate is quite small from pro vitamin A.

Fermentation and Vegetables

Let's take sauerkraut as a convenient example because most people will be familiar with it. Sauerkraut is fermented cabbage.

From the German language 'sauer' means 'sour', and 'kraut' means 'cabbage'. The Germans were also called 'Krauts' during the war, because of their love for eating the stuff. Now, like all vegetables, cabbage contains small amounts of poison as a defence against insects. In the case of cabbage, the primary poison is Oxalic acid. This is an irritant to humans too, which is why we cook the cabbage (generally) before eating it. The other way of reducing the oxalic acid is to ferment the cabbage. There's a natural bacterium that lives on the cabbage and it will happily consume the oxalic acid and turn it into useful products like acetic acid and lactic acid. This takes time though; approximately one to six months for the fermentation to bring out the potential of the cabbage. Fermentation, which is breeding up the bacteria, unlocks the vitamins from the cabbage. For example, a cup of cabbage probably contains around 30mg of vitamin C. A cup of Sauerkraut will contain 600mg of vitamin C. Aren't those bacteria clever?

If you're looking at making, or eating sauerkraut, to assist your health or Depression, then I'd encourage you to do so. You don't have to stop at sauerkraut though, you can ferment just about anything; carrots, beets, eggs, asparagus, garlic, fish, etc.

The point is that vegetables are good, don't get me wrong, but fermented vegetables are an absolute power-house of nutrition. Remember, raw and cooked vegetables alone, are not what humans were designed to eat.

Well, I'm getting to the end of this chapter and so far, it sounds like a rant against vegetarians and vegans, but there is a purpose beyond that. I have vegetarian friends who are pleasant and not depressed. If you've made it this far, you'll know that I strongly believe Depression is caused by poor gut health and poor food choices. I'm just trying to say that if you're a vegetarian, it can be really hard to obtain the right oils and the right vitamins from your food. If you suffer with Depression, I'd encourage you to put your vegetarianism aside until the Depression is gone. If you wish to go back to it later, then that's fine. Failing that, get some quality, fermented vegetables into you, they're a massive source of vitamins, bacteria and fibre. Don't make the mistake of fermenting for a few days, or only a week, like I did. It just isn't enough time, and the stuff will irritate your gut, rather than heal it.

Plants and Poisons

Every single plant including edible vegetables and fruits, contain a small amount of poison. This is nature's chemical weapon against insect attack. That juicy orange tree or spinach plant has the same goal as every other life form: to grow and reproduce. Being eaten is not on its agenda. Now some seeds do actually want to be eaten, so they spread themselves around, but basically speaking, the skin of fruit is designed to protect the seeds and stop them from being eaten.

In relation to an orange for example, the thin, orange, outer layer is there to attract bees for pollination. The thick pith is created to protect the flesh from insects. The pith is usually bitter and that's why we don't eat it. It's also a physical barrier to insects. The flesh is food to nourish the seeds, and the seeds themselves contain cyanide, which is probably why we don't eat them.

You can do a google search on any plant food you eat and you'll find that it contains a poison or irritant. In the case of rhubarb, we don't eat the leaves. They contain the highest amount of oxalic acid, which is irritating to the gut. After you trim the leaves off, cook the shit out of it ... that removes most of the remaining oxalic acid. With rice, the poison is arsenic; in wheat, it's gluten, and in Quinoa, the poison is saponins. For potatoes and tomatoes, it's lectins; for almonds, its cyanide. Basmati rice is the most prized rice of all, why? It has the lowest arsenic content.

With all these foods, they can be eaten, but they should be properly prepared. To eat an orange, first remove the peel and don't eat the seeds. With rice, boil it, throw away the water, and rinse it. Pumpkin; remove the skin and seeds and boil thoroughly. Italian tinned tomatoes are usually beautiful because the Italians normally skin and de-seed the tomatoes. This process removes almost all of the lectins. Absolutely every plant-based food has something in it that's annoying, so it just makes sense to limit your exposure to these poisons. The 'traditional way' of preparing these foods is generally the best. The traditional methods of preparation have faced thousands of years of scrutiny, so it's just easy to ignore them for the sake of expediency. My point again is that vegetarianism can be done, and successfully, but you have to be careful about it, because it is not the natural order of things.

Just before I end this chapter…found the following article, which seems to sum up what I'm saying. You might want to take a look at:

'The Baffling Connection Between Vegetarianism and Depression'.
(Web Source: https://www.psychologytoday.com/au/blog/animals-and-us/201812/)

In Defence of Vegetarians

There is a defence. Fruit and vegetables contain the most amount of dietary fibre of any foods. Dietary fibre is super important to feed gut bacteria. That's why the CSIRO amongst others recommends 5 serves of vegetables per day. I suggest that their recommendations are correct, they just don't state why they are correct. They are correct because of the high fibre content is needed to feed your gut bacteria.

Nuts, (not peanuts but real nuts) contain many beneficial compounds and oils. Grains and beans I am not so hot on because of the indigestible proteins found like lectins and gluten. Beans and grains are fine if they are handled properly like by vigorous cooking or fermentation. Apparently its healthy today to "activate" the nuts you eat, like almonds for example. You activate the nuts, mostly by soaking them. Activating them is a nice term, but it really means soaking them to remove the poisons. The poison in almonds (for example) is cyanide. Of course with modern almonds, most (but not all) of the cyanide has been bred out.

The thing is veggos, the cultivation of green leafy and above ground vegetables is in evolutionary terms, quite new. The accepted timeline for cultivation of crops is about 10,000 years. The accepted timeline for the existence of humans (homo sapiens) is 150,000 years. In other words, vegetables only showed up yesterday."

Root vegetables like yams, carrots, parsnip, ginger, and cassava (which doesn't include potatoes) have been with us forever it would seem. The point is, green leafy vegetables obviously can be eaten, though they are new to the diet, so you should to be a bit careful about these new foods. Good, old-fashioned root vegetables contain immense amounts of dietary fibre. Eat plenty of them...just don't forget that healthy fats, proteins and vitamins are found mainly in meat.

I've seen studies recommending various amounts of meat and animal products in the diet, ranging from 10% meat to 100% meat. These diets claim to be the 'healthiest'. I don't know which is best, but they all contain some meat. Obviously, there are those espousing the vegetarian and vegan diet as being the healthiest too. The point is that if you think about it in historical and evolutionary terms, a diet without animal products is not the natural order of things. By all means eat a heavily vegetable diet, but don't forget the meat if you want to be really healthy.

Handout to Veggos

If I was only faced with farmed fish and factory-produced cow meat, I'd be tempted to go veggo too! The meat industry has done enormous damage to itself by breeding cows, chickens, and fish in concentration camp like conditions. They also feed the animals un-natural diets in crowded environments. The meat of today just isn't real meat. Likewise, hydroponic lettuces and kale are possibly worthless vegetables. The conditions many animals endure today do very little for our nutrition or our environment.

Veggos, I understand your outrage...it is justified. Unfortunately for you, monocrop, artificially fertilised vegetables are equally at fault. There are alternatives though. Sustainably raised meat and fish are great sources of calories and nutrition. I'd like to say the same about vegetables, but they're hard to find too. Go for naturalness is all I can suggest. You'll be rewarded in terms of your mental and physical health.

CHAPTER 14

In Praise of Alcohol

Let me start with a disclaimer. Don't you hate them? It's not a big one, and you've probably heard it before. "Overindulgence in alcohol will make your Depression worse."

I believe this is universally accepted but occasional overindulgence, with periods of abstinence, may be fine. What I want to discuss are some of the benefits of moderate alcohol consumption.

Some people think of drinking alcohol as 'morally the wrong thing to do' or 'bad for one's health'. These people feel the same way about eating meat, salt consumption, sugar intake, and probably the sun. If you look at the statistics you'll find the countries with the highest alcohol consumption, and those who eat the most meat, salt, and sugar, are the most desirable countries to live in. They also have the highest incomes, and live the longest lives. Is there a message there? Hopefully there is. I mean take Saudi Arabia for example, where alcohol is outlawed. There's hardly a conga line of immigrants dying to get in, despite their high per capita income. I note that life expectancy in Saudi has improved over the last fifty years, but it remains approximately ten years less than highly developed countries in the west, like the USA, or Switzerland.

Now it could easily be said that this is due to other factors, and that's possibly the case but everyone loves to look for some other cause.

Maybe, just maybe, increased alcohol consumption isn't a result of increased wealth or stress. Perhaps it works the other way round. As in, increased alcohol consumption leads to increased wealth, or a higher standard of living. Sounds heretical right? Well how do we know? The answer is…we don't. And perhaps moderate alcohol consumption makes people smarter, happier, and more productive. I've certainly had times in my life, following moderate alcohol consumption, when I've been happier. I may have felt smarter too, but that might be delusional. 'Smartness' might be like beauty; in the eye of the beholder. Being more productive following alcohol consumption, I don't know about that one, but it seems doubtful. Still, I do know this from first-hand experience. My tennis game is much better following a beer or two. One can of beer is about the limit of the effect. The reason: alcohol induces relaxation. Beyond that one beer, for me, my reaction times start to slow too much. I even have a mate who checks to ensure I've had a drink before a match. If not, he won't be my doubles partner because he knows we'll lose. So, in that regard, light alcohol consumption does make me more productive. I'm not suggesting this at an elite athlete level, or for endurance sports. Most of us don't dwell there though.

My father was a roof tile maker, the boss of a company. When he visited a factory in Germany, everyone stopped for morning tea and the beer cart came around. Most workers had one beer, which is usually a good-sized portion in Germany. No one went crazy and had too many. My father said to the boss, "if I did this at home, I wouldn't get anyone back to work." The German boss replied, "If I didn't do this, no one would go back to work." And this was a very large, successful company.

I was recently at what I regard as the 'world's best Airport'. It's Munich. Around 7am, we reached the gate. Everyone in the family was hungry so we went and hunted down breakfast. The reason I class Munich as the world's best Airport is because you can have a litre of the world's best beer with your breakfast, which is surprisingly popular. I refrained as I try to restrict my drinking until after breakfast, but then again, I am a bit of a prude. There were no drunks or fights in this place, and everything runs on time. If you don't get a beer with your bacon, there's no reason for despair…you can get a small can (half a litre) from the newsagency to drink while reading your newspaper. You don't have to drink the world's best beer either; they have imported brands as well.

Just in case you were wondering if Munich might be a bit backward or unproductive, it's the home of BMW, the 'B' being Bavaria, a state of Germany; Munich as the capital. Audi is about 45 minutes drive from the capital, and VW's about the same. Mercedes Benz and Porsche are just up the road. Apparently, Munich is also the most expensive real estate in Germany. I know it's just an anecdote, but ones like this require attention. I'll take an anecdote every day, over a scientific study. Munich workers are serious about their alcohol consumption, and seriously productive as well. Under German law, beer isn't even classified as an alcoholic beverage; it's classified as a food.

So, the point I'm making is that moderate alcohol consumption can easily be linked to the most desirable, and sometimes the most productive places to live. Things may start going astray if you consume distilled (concentrated) spirits on a regular basis, but sticking to beer and wine seems to work. In fact, if I plotted a graph of wine and beer consumption vs longevity, or vs per capita income, I reckon I'd find a very close correlation. It's quite difficult to do; I'd have to make some adjustment for the average amount of alcohol in each drink, like 5% for beer and 12.5% for wine. The countries that consistently come up in statistics as being the top consumers are: Germany, France, Australia, Sweden, Holland, England, USA, and Switzerland. They all have high incomes, high standards of living, and desirable destinations for immigrants.

Countries that rank lowly include Pakistan, Bangladesh, Yemen, Egypt, and Afghanistan. They are also the least desirable countries for immigration.

Alcohol gets such a bad wrap these days that it's about time someone stood up for it.

One of the big problems with alcohol now (same as the food supply) is all the preservatives, packaging, and process 'improvements' that make the drinks less 'natural'. This is why the Germans can get away with what they do, because of the strict regulations on beer in particular. German beer is just about the most natural you can get, unless you brew it yourself. By the way… it's sort of a side issue, but fermenting sugar and water has a tendency to purify the water. Before chlorine was invented, yeast and bacteria were used to 'purify' water, making it fit to drink. We still do it today; sewage farms use bacteria to purify water before discharging it. Those bacteria aren't alcohol-producing bacteria though. Just as well, otherwise fish would get drunk, as well as poisoned.

Prohibition

There's only ever been one properly conducted experiment on banning alcohol in a democratic country, to my knowledge. That was prohibition in the USA from 1920 to 1933.

It's widely accepted that the per capita consumption of alcohol didn't change much, except for the extreme ends. People who drank a lot probably drank more, and people who hardly drank at all, probably drank less. Everyone in-between probably remained about the same. Naturally, it's hard to obtain accurate statistics when the industry is driven underground.

There was definitely an increase in organised crime. These crims suddenly found a new source of income with a strong, diverse market. There was also a big loss in government revenue. In fact, it would appear the deficit was a massive driver behind abolishing prohibition. The Great Depression that began in 1929 caused such a severe loss in government revenue that it needed to be replaced somehow. The government basically decided to take taxes from alcohol in order to run the country. Maybe prohibition contributed to The Great Depression somehow. I know I'd be pretty depressed if I couldn't legally have a drink for thirteen years!

People say this jokingly now: "I'm just having this alcohol for medicinal purposes." I've worked out the origin of this saying. During prohibition, the only people who could dispense alcohol legally were pharmacists. They also required a doctor's prescription for it. The number of prescriptions prescribed for alcohol went through the roof and alcohol sales through the pharmacy/drug stores did too. In fact, a number of doctors were caught selling prescriptions to organised crime gangs. But in all seriousness, alcohol does induce a therapeutic effect. Like any medicine, one can overdose, but when used wisely, alcohol is a force for good.

I mean everyone wants to get back to nature and put natural products in their body. Wine and beer for example, are completely natural. I'll tell you what isn't natural: Diet Coke, blue Gatorade, Ice cream, French Fries, hydroponic lettuce and Kale, refrigerators, aeroplanes, nylon clothes, vitamin tablets, boost juice (blended at 15000 rpm), Stevia (concentrated 400 times) and coconut oil (who was the clever dick that decided to make oil from those nuts).

Natural Wine

As usual, I digress. Alcohol, particularly wine, is one of the most natural products you can get. It isn't cooked, refined, or concentrated. It's just the result of completely natural processes. Grow some grapes. Crush them in your hands, or have virgins stomp on them (even non-virgins will do, since virgins are a rare commodity), stick the juice in a container and let it sit in the dark for a few weeks. There you have it ... wine. Apparently, too much sugar is bad for you and I probably support that notion. If you allow the wine to ferment properly, the sugar will all be gone. The wine is way healthier for you than the grape juice it was made from. I mean now that we've industrialised the process of winemaking, there's certainly some stuff in it that's un-natural. We should be blaming the winemaking process, plus the fact that we buy the junk, not the alcohol itself per se. I have this one criticism of most modern wine: its high alcohol content. If you go back fifty, even a hundred years ago, you'll find that common wine contained a lower alcohol content. Today, due to the use of modern yeasts, their availability, and processing methods, wine typically has concentrations of 13-15% alcohol. This makes the wine too strong and that's why beer is a much better option, containing about 5% alcohol.

Special Groups

If you're an Asian person or an Australian Aboriginal, you have to be a little more careful of alcohol. This possibly includes Native Americans as well, I'm not too sure. Reason being, you're likely to be lacking in an enzyme called 'alcohol dehydrogenase'. My suspicion is that this enzyme can be built up, but only by drinking the right type of alcohol. The wrong type is anything made from wheat, grain, or concentrates. The Japanese drink rice wine, or Sake. I suspect this may work for them, but again, Japanese people need to be extra careful. I'd say that any good quality wine would work for just about anyone. By good quality, I don't mean expensive. The stuff I drink costs around $20 per litre, and it's organic. I drink too much of it, and I haven't suffered from a hangover in years.

Alcohol 'Can Be' Your Friend

I sincerely hope dear readers that you do drink alcohol for its therapeutic benefits. Use it wisely and it will be your friend. Thing is, if you don't drink alcohol, then your body will make it for you. The bacteria and yeast in your system, naturally, will produce tiny amounts of alcohol all the time, day and night, whether you want it to occur, or not. It too has calming and therapeutic benefits. When you kill off your natural bacteria with antibiotics and toxic, un-natural chemicals and foods, you limit the ability for your body to produce the alcohol that's good for your health. I know I'm pushing the envelope here, but alcohol is a bit like cholesterol; it's good for your health, up to a point. If your body doesn't receive it as in food or drink, then it will be forced to make it, and your body isn't happy about that...it uses up too much energy.

In my humble opinion, alcohol saved my life when I was suffering with Depression. If I wasn't drinking at the time, I don't think I'd have been able to function. Maybe I would have 'done myself in' - sadly lots of people do. Those on the outside of Depression like to give you advice, but honestly, they have no idea what it's like on the inside. Perhaps if we just administered a small amount of alcohol to Depression sufferers, their mental health would improve. Even if it didn't, maybe their survival rate would be higher. It's pretty hard to 'do yourself in' if you're drunk all the time, unless you're doing something foolish like driving a car or using a chainsaw. Maybe the reason I was a 'high functioning' person with Depression, was because I consumed alcohol on almost a daily basis.

Staying alive is the only thing that really matters. If that means having a few drinks every day, then go for it. It's way better to be alive and drunk any day, in preference to the alternative. Obviously being alive and sober is the pinnacle, but Depression sucks, and if you need a few drinks to endure it, then I say do it...just don't overdo it (and that's easy to do).

The Downsides

During the course of writing this book, I admit to having a short relapse of Depression. I suspect this was primarily caused by an over-indulgence of alcohol, repeated over several months. Though it did help me further discover some of the mechanisms of alcohol, serotonin, and digestion. I mean it's a hell of a way to find this out. Basically, moderate alcohol consumption will increase your serotonin production, which is a good thing if you're depressed.

You just have to be careful about overdoing it, and don't do it all the time. When your body repeatedly has its serotonin boosted by alcohol, then it turns down its formation of natural serotonin. This is most likely a strong cause of alcoholism: Serotonin production is turned down by repeated alcohol ingestion, so you crave more alcohol to make the serotonin back, and the cycle repeats. Hangovers are most likely made worse by the depletion of serotonin, after drinking too much. Then some people have a 'hair of the dog', which is a short-term boost to serotonin.

There are many other dark sides to alcohol consumption, as we all know. Most of them come from over-indulgence. Studies however, reveal the health benefits of moderate to low alcohol consumption, and my belief is that this applies to Depression sufferers also. In fact, I just read a study in today's paper showing that moderate alcohol consumption appears to have a protective effect from Dementia. (Moderate = 14 drinks per week, for the average male).

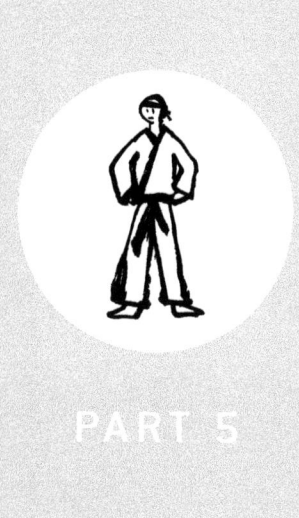

PART 5

FOOD + MEDICINE

CHAPTER 15

Concentration + Commoditisation

Concentration sort of Fucks Everything Up!

When you concentrate something, the tendency is to fuck it. And the most concentrated thing that you probably have in your kitchen right now is sugar. We've all been told how bad it is, right? Well sugar is only a 10x concentrate. In other words, ten tonnes of sugar cane = one tonne of sugar.

Ten times isn't a big deal really... what about a concentrate that's 100x, 400x or 1000x. Do you know what's concentrated 400x? Stevia. Know what else? Cocaine; it's 400x as well. Heroin is 1000x.

There's not that much wrong with sugar. Sugar cane is actually a superfood. It's a complete food if you eat the inner part of the plant, including the fibre. You'd receive plenty of vitamins, minerals and fibre, plus a good helping of sugar. But when you concentrate it, strip out the fibre, minerals, and vitamins, it becomes dead calories, and that's what you get in a lot of foods today. So, we try to add the vitamins and minerals back into it. But we forget to add the fibre as well. And do the vitamins and minerals that are added back in, work as well as the original?

By the way, this chapter isn't about sugar or sugar substitutes, I'm just using some examples of concentrates here.

Stevia

I don't recommend Stevia, or any other sugar substitutes, but let's talk about it. Stevia is not Stevia. What does this mean?

Stevia is a green, leafy plant that you can grow in your backyard.

If you want to use those leaves in your coffee, I have no objection. They won't sweeten your coffee much though. If you want to sweeten your coffee, you'll need to concentrate it about 400x.

On one of the Stevia product websites, I read that Stevia is distilled in a natural steam distillation process. What does that mean? Can anyone think of a natural source of steam? Oh, okay yes, a volcano. So grab your leaves and hold them over a vent hole in the volcano…good luck with that! And…you'll need a natural distillation column. This would assumedly be made from natural stainless steel. You'll also have to install it using a natural, 10-tonne crane. Are you kidding me?

There's no such thing as a natural steam distillation process. You could be waiting somewhere between ten, and a million years, for the natural steam to rise from the volcano. Basically, 'controlled steam' was only invented a few hundred years ago.

Anyway, disposing of that argument, I'm not against steam distillation, I just object to the alleged 'naturalness' of it. Anyway, now we have 400kg of Stevia leaf and distil it to produce 1kg of Stevia sweetener.

Hopefully there aren't any nasties in there, because we'll possibly concentrate them 400 times as well. I'm willing to accept it's free of gremlins, and let's say it's pure Stevia Glycosides.

The other day I was looking through my local supermarket for products labelled 'STEVIA'. The first one I came across was '50% not Stevia'. I was shocked. The label clearly stated 'Stevia' but only half (or less) was actually Stevia, the main ingredient was glucose. So if we compare this to table sugar, it's 50% glucose as well: no different.

I then checked two other Stevia products. Both had large labels with the prominent word 'Stevia'. They contained '99.6% <u>not</u> Stevia'. In other words, the Stevia content was 0.4% or less. The remaining 99.6% is often sugar, glucose, or erythritol (a sugar alcohol).

I told my wife and when she checked the following day, another product was found, also labelled 'Stevia'. This one contained 99.7% sugar and 0.3% Stevia (stevia extract). The claim was that you could use 50% less of the product, because it 'tastes so much sweeter' due to the Stevia extract.

So, if it were possible (and it's not) to concentrate cane sugar 400x, instead of 10x, you'd also have a product that's very sweet and low in calories, but would you do it?

Take cocaine leaves (Coca leaves) for example. If you live in Columbia, you can just pick a couple of leaves on your way to work and chew them, equivalent to us here in Australia, or the USA, drinking our morning cup of coffee? It gives us a mild buzz and relaxes us for the day, no big deal, right?

But when you shove a pound of leaves up your nose, it has a vastly different effect. It would be like having four hundred cups of coffee before work, or maybe forty cans of Red Bull.

Even pure Stevia powder, if you can find it, is a highly refined product, nothing like the original source. I'd avoid it if possible.

I've always experienced gut or respiratory side effects with Stevia. Maybe you don't, but are you looking for it? Are you just using it because it's not-sugar and you think that sugar's bad for you? Perhaps you want to lower your calorie intake for weight reasons, or because it's the 'trendy' thing to do. I'm not having a go at you, I'm just suggesting you think about what you're doing, because substituting a bit of sugar with a bit of poison, isn't always the answer.

Just as an aside, I like Rapadura sugar. It's dehydrated sugar cane juice, so it contains loads of minerals. It has a distinct flavour though. I suspect it's more like an 8x or 9x concentrate.

Making Coca Leaf into Cocaine

Reagents required: Kerosene Solid Na_2CO_3 Distilled H_2O H_2SO_4 5% Solid $KMnO_4$ (6% Solution is used) NH_4OH 10% HCl 37% Acetone Diethyl Ether.

Do you really want to shove that up your nose? It might be okay every now and then, but I wouldn't know... never done it. Lack of opportunity probably. The thing is, taking stuff like Stevia is voluntary, and you do it to yourself every day, because sugar is so awful. I'd take sugar every day, over Stevia. Coca leaf is probably fine too, if you just chew a few leaves each day. I don't know about the concentrated product though.

It's all about Concentration

Olive oil:	3kg olives	=	1kg olive oil
Soya bean oil:	8kg soya beans	=	1 litre soy oil
Canola oil:	2.5kg canola seeds	=	1 litre canola oil
Sunflower oil:	1.5kg sunflower seeds	=	1kg sunflower oil.

The further difference between these oils is the degree of processing required. Going back a hundred years, there was no way you could make soya bean oil, sunflower, or canola (even if they existed). These oils absolutely rely on modern hydraulic presses, and processing methods. Olive oil has likely been around for thousands of years. The others... maybe fifty years, so we have no idea of their true health effects.

1 orange	=	75mg vitamin C
1 Vitamin C tablet	=	1000mg vitamin C
14 oranges	=	1 x 1000mg vitamin C tablet (except that Vitamin C is rarely made from oranges. Usually, it's made from petrol).

If you're eating anything that didn't exist a hundred years ago, and consuming concentrates, you're asking for trouble in my opinion. Sure, we can run all kinds of tests to prove this stuff isn't harmful in the short term, but I'd like to see some testing ran over a course of fifty to a hundred years. They'd be answers worth listening to.

Vitamin Tablets

All vitamins are a concentrate. Most of them aren't even made from the foods they're naturally found in, but that's not the point. Just take the vitamin C from above: 1000mg of vitamin C, delivered at once in a tiny, concentrated form. How does your body deal with it? I'm not saying that I know the answer, but when you think about it, it's quite a big ask. To swallow fourteen oranges at once, with no dilution, and expect that our systems will naturally cope with it, is not something that has occurred in evolutionary history. I've heard that people who take vitamins recognise that much of what they take, is excreted in their urine. They don't seem to mind, I suppose at least some of it sticks. The thing is that your body has to somehow cope with a concentrated substance that it's never dealt with before. All concentrates are worth paying attention to. That isn't to say they're all poison, but they could be, so you should be careful.

Be sceptical of anything that's in a concentrated form.

What does this mean to People Fighting Depression?

It means that I'm trying to give you a fighting chance of beating this chronic condition. Just because something is deemed 'natural' or 'organic', doesn't mean it's good for you. There's an awful lot of heroin around, and that's organic and natural...but it doesn't mean it's good for you. On the other hand, if you consumed an entire opium flower, it might possibly be okay, because you're getting the whole package, as nature intended. I don't know the answer to that, again, I've never tried it, but I suspect you wouldn't get high.

What I do know is that when I was a young guy, I smoked plenty of Marijuana. I inhaled deeply and got high. Somewhere along the line, a 'new' hydroponic form of Marijuana was introduced. The stuff was strong, and it certainly got you high, but it was awful. The experience was an intense, crazy high…not the mellow 'who gives a toss' kind of high. All of the 'bad' elements from getting high were concentrated; paranoia, the 'munchies', and negative thoughts.

I suspect the vast majority of you have experienced alcohol at some stage. I certainly hope so, as it's one of my favourite pleasures in life. So, in yourself, do you notice a difference between drinking rum, or a good quality red wine? Of course you do. Rum makes you crazy and aggressive, whereas red wine makes you mellow and reflective. I'm not the first person to discover this. There's a scientific reason behind it. It's all about the concentration, and processing. Wine is more or less, as nature intended it to be. Rum is a highly refined and concentrated product. Once you refine and concentrate a product, as I said earlier, there's a great tendency to fuck it up. This doesn't mean that all rum is bad, it just means that 'badly made rum' is bad.

Not only Concentration, but Commoditisation

Commoditisation tends to fuck everything as well.

The term basically comes from the word 'commodity', meaning something is sold into the marketplace in large quantities, based on its weight or volume. The quality of the product is usually sacrificed. Last year we found a source of heritage breed, 'properly fed chickens' for consumption. They were hard to find. These chickens are totally delectable. They have much smaller bones, less fat, and really tasty meat. A 2kg chicken will feed a family of five with plenty of leftovers. The chickens are around $30 each (not cheap), but the satisfaction and taste is just so much better, and the entire family enjoys the experience. You'll probably struggle to find them in your local area. Regular chickens for purchase in your supermarket, are commoditised. Even free range and organic chickens are commoditised. I'm not telling you to do what I do, that requires some work and investigation. But I strongly suggest you go for quality over quantity, and your life will get better.

When things are commoditised, just like concentration, it tends to fuck them. Not all concentrations are bad though, neither are all commodities. But the tendency is to sacrifice the good bits, and to sacrifice the quality.

If you're depressed, I say spend whatever money you can on yourself, indulge, and go for quality. Fact is; you'll pay, one way or another. You could spend years chasing commoditised medicines and food, waste a lot of precious time, or just indulge yourself with quality food and wine. You'll end up in the same place either way, except you'll be older, with or without Depression. Better to be older without it, I say.

Coconut Oil is a Commodity

Let me super digress here just for a minute and talk about coconut oil. This is a modern super food apparently.

The islanders of let's say Samoa, five hundred years ago, used coconuts for just about everything. But do you think they looked at one and said, "hey, you know what? I'll gather fifty coconuts and pound the shit out of them to make oil for our hair. Or we could make candles out of it, even cook the pig in it." I'm telling you, these guys had better things to do with their time. They made better use of their limited calories and energy as well. I'm willing to believe that coconut oil may have been used as a medicine, but our bodies weren't made to digest it. Coconut oil didn't exist until it became a commodity. So what you're doing is experimenting. Having said that, I'm pretty sure coconut oil is reasonably healthy and way better than soy bean, sunflower, or canola oil, all of which are even more recent developments.

The experiment that has been running for thousands, perhaps millions of years, shows that people kill and eat animals. They cook and eat them as quickly as they can, before other predators and scavengers move in and take it away. I'm sorry if this sounds a bit brutal.

Something else is important here: There were few carbohydrates or sugars in the diet until about 10,000 years ago. Sugar/fruit was only an occasional delicacy.

If you've been following the theme of this book, you'll understand that I'm suggesting you eat and put things in your body, in the way your body was designed to receive them. You have to try and think to some extent, like a caveman. It will give you the greatest chance to solve issues of Depression.

Meat is a Commodity and a Concentrate

You'll know from earlier reading that I love eating meat. With factory-farmed and feedlot animals, they too are a commodity and a concentrate. The animals aren't fed their natural diet. They exist far from a natural environment. "That's fair enough, so just change to grass-fed meat." That's a good first step.

It's the concentration that I want to concentrate on…ha ha! No seriously, it's the fact that we only eat the muscle meat. We should eat the entire animal.

Meat should be eaten with all the fat included, or at least cooked with it all attached. Just try it once and you'll see what I mean about the flavour aspect. It doesn't end there though. What you should eat (and I don't) is all of the animal. That's what made ancient people's diets so nutrient and vitamin dense. Modern people basically eat the muscle meat of the beast. According to legend, the North American Indians threw the muscle meat to their dogs (that's the part we eat). The Indians themselves went for the thyroid gland, the heart, liver, and brains of their captured prey. They sort of fought over the 'good bits.'

Take my word for it; ancient civilisations ate the entire animal from head to tail. Some of it raw, some frozen, most of it roasted (they didn't have a pot), and ate all of the organs. What I like to do now is eat the occasional organ, but you have to prepare it well, otherwise it tastes like shit. If you ate cow's liver every now and then, or steak tartare, it would be great for your health. I don't judge you if you don't want to, but you should eat like your grandparents ate, even if it's only occasionally.

In regards to beef, one of the most highly sought-after types of beef is wagyu. It's judged by how 'marbled' it is. Marbling is the fat that's dispersed through the muscle meat. That adds flavour. The real point I want to focus on though is that fat should not be dispersed through the muscle. Muscle should be muscle, surrounded by fat. The fat should be on the outside of the muscle, as it is in your own body. We manipulate the diet of wagyu beef cattle, by feeding them an unnatural diet. It tastes fantastic, and I'm not against eating it. All we're really doing is hiding the fat from our eyes, but it's still there. I personally have no trouble with fat, invisible or not. I'm quite certain that within fifty years we'll come to respect fat again, and its importance in our diet. And we'll also appreciate that an occasional serving of liver is far cheaper and healthier than a vitamin tablet. Hey, I don't often have a raw liver shake, but I should. If I told you that you could solve your Depression by consuming a raw liver shake (a completely legal product) once a week, would you do it? Again, I don't have your answer, but please think about it. You're not going to die from it, and it may well make you feel a whole lot better.

All I'm saying is, be careful. Spend a bit more time thinking about your food choices and try to get your food in the most natural and unprocessed way that you can. Like Hippocrates said, *"Let food be thy Medicine."*

CHAPTER 16

Natural vs Unnatural

I'm pretty sure most of us know the difference between what's natural and unnatural. Anything that wasn't invented until the last hundred years is probably unnatural. The problem is, in my opinion, we're much too lenient.

If something comes from nature, isn't poisonous, or contains nutrition, then we tend to accept it as natural. But let's just examine a few examples to show you why we're too easy-going.

Take a carrot … what colour is it? (I gather most of you will say 'orange').

Actually, to my knowledge there are at least a hundred varieties of carrots, and most of them aren't orange. The type that we grow now, come from less than ten common varieties. The 'orange' carrot was only developed around five hundred years ago; a gift from plant breeders in Holland to commemorate their Dutch King, whose colours are orange. I'm not saying carrots aren't good for you, or that they're unnatural, but you should beware of your acceptance of things that are natural. If I'd asked this question five hundred years ago, the answer would likely have been purple, green, or white. So when you selectively breed carrots to be orange (always), you're essentially taking 'self-selection' away from the plant, to be a different colour. In the case of carrots, purple carrots contain anthocyanins, which are apparently good for your health. (The red/purple colour comes from beneficial anthocyanins). They are not present in modern, orange carrots.

When you buy a zucchini, it is sold by weight. The wholesaler also buys it by weight. For farmers to gain maximum profit, they need to increase the plants' weight just before harvest. This means getting as much water into it as possible, without killing it. In turn, the water also dilutes the calories and nutrients. Therefore, by weight, the zucchini is far less nutritious than it used to be. The zucchini will be at its maximum nutrient density just as it ripens, and should be picked and freshly eaten at that time. But we simply can't do that in our modern world because it would likely rot on the way to market. So, it must be harvested before it reaches its full potential. Here's an easy fix: Buy the smallest, greenest zucchinis you can get, they will be more nutrient dense. A hundred years ago, large zucchinis probably didn't exist because rabbits or insects would eat them before they reached maturity. So I'm saying that those huge zucchinis are probably far 'less natural' than you think.

Oranges

I love those beautiful, juicy Sunkist oranges from California. They look fantastic too. Most people would consider them to be full of natural goodness. They probably are. As I live in Australia, I estimate that a Sunkist orange would be picked at least two months before I'm fortunate enough to eat one. It has to be harvested, stored, packed, transported to a warehouse, loaded onto a ship (they don't fly them out, do they?), shipped to Australia, put in another warehouse, distributed from the port to central distribution, then trucked to my supermarket. I'm exhausted just thinking about it. Then it sits on the shelf for a few more days, waiting for me to buy it. I take it home, and if it's lucky, it will be eaten sometime within the following week. There's just no way in the world that 'this' orange can be as nutritious as the one I grow in my backyard. I don't grow oranges by the way, but you know what I mean. I've seen various estimates on vitamin C content and how it degrades with time. I've also read about comparisons between a 'natural, hand-picked orange' eaten straight from the tree, and a store-bought orange that has been in transit for months. There's a massive drop in Vitamin C content between the tree orange and the supermarket orange.

Milk

Milk is one of the most mucked-about products on the market. The dairy cow breed used in Australia is Friesian Holstein, or Holstein. These cows are used to get the maximum milk production, not the best quality milk. These animals are somewhat of a compromise. The best quality milk with the highest butterfat content is produced by Guernsey, or Jersey cows. Using Holsteins again relates directly to farmers' profitability and has little to do with your health. If you homogenise the milk, or reduce the fat, you are further compromising an already compromised product.

If you want to find out how they make low fat milk, Google it. You'll be surprised what you're drinking, and how it has been handled. It isn't just regular milk with a bit of fat skimmed off.

Pure, clean, unpasteurised milk from a cow is almost as nutritious as mothers' milk for a newborn baby. You just can't get that kind of milk today unless you live on a farm and milk Jersey or Guernsey cows. I'm not suggesting you don't drink milk…but buy a type that has been mucked-about with the least. The more processing they do, the further from nature you get.

Sunflower

It's just like the coconut oil we talked about earlier. Who looks at a sunflower and says, "Hey, I'll make some cooking oil out of that?" The whole process relies on modern agriculture, mechanical harvesting, huge hydraulic presses and extraction methods. If you call that natural, then I'm okay with that, but it's a bit far-fetched.

Wheat

Here are a couple of fun facts about wheat. Most wheat grown (in Australia anyway) is called Dwarf wheat. It grows about 3ft high and has a huge head with lots of seeds. Going back fifty years, the wheat was more like 5ft tall with fewer seeds. More energy went into the stalk, and less into the seeds. Dwarf wheat also has a higher gluten content and something like thirty chromosomes. Before that, wheat only contained fourteen chromosomes. Does that make a difference to your health? I don't know, but it might.

When you have a hundred acres of wheat to harvest, you book a harvesting contractor to harvest it for you. He's booked in on a certain date. As a farmer, you need the wheat ready to be harvested on that day, to get the maximum yield. All the wheat has to be 'ripe' on that date too. So what do they do? Spray it with 'Roundup' (weed killer). This helps ripen the wheat so it's ready for when the harvester arrives. Then the farmer gets the best yield. Does spraying it with Roundup enhance its nutritional qualities? I'm not sure, but I doubt it. Do you want your wheat to be sprayed with weed poison before you eat it? I can't answer that question for you either (but I know I don't). Does the poison end up in your food? I don't know, I just prefer not to have to wonder. I don't claim that Roundup causes cancer, Depression, or any health concern. I just prefer to eliminate it, out of an abundance of caution.

All wheat flour in Australia, USA, Canada, and the UK, is fortified with folic acid (except organic wheat). Folic acid is a synthetic version of vitamin B9. Is that good or bad? I don't know, but it's not natural. Folic acid has only existed for around seventy-five years. And supplements are made in a factory. I absolutely guarantee, there aren't trucks full of spinach, lined up at the gates of the folic acid factory. They're not waiting to offload their cargo for the factory to make folic acid out of it. So even 'natural' wheat may be far less natural than you think. Now obviously modern wheat doesn't cause Depression, or everyone would have it.

The thing is, <u>you</u> my dear reader, may be suffering from Depression. I doubt that eating organic wheat will fix that situation. Again, I'm just trying to give you the best chance of fixing it. It's not that hard to change something like your wheat source.

Look... I'm not trying to paint a bleak picture, really. I'm just warning you not to be fooled by all the claims of so-called natural substances that can help you. Especially when it comes to health and Depression. Be a bit critical of what you put in your mouth and try to buy things that are as natural as possible, without obsessing about it. As I've said before, you can only do the best you can when it comes to being as 'natural' as possible. And try to eat a fully naturally-derived meal as often as you can.

Natural Chicken

Chickens are a great example of natural versus unnatural. I've devised a table in regard to the relative nutritional goodness of a chicken.

Lets take a regular battery-fed chicken as the base, and give it a score of 1. This chicken has spent its entire life in a tiny portion of a shed where low light from artificial sources shines down for 23 hours of the day. It only eats pellets made from the cheapest products, which provide the bird with a maximum growth rate. These chickens are carefully selected breeds with the fastest growth-to-calorific input ratio. So for all the hundreds of breeds of chickens, the battery-fed variety is selected for rapid growth and minimum input; nothing to do with its nutritional content, or flavour.

The next breed we'll examine is the free-range chicken. This bird is exactly the same as the battery-fed variety (also a score of 1). The only difference between the two is that this chicken has a small hole cut out of its cage to allow it to roam around in the space between the chicken sheds. In other words, it can go outside if it wants to. The area between these sheds is barren; no food or sunshine, so hardly different to the environment inside the cage. The average time this chicken spends outside of its cage is only a small part of its life. Maybe every now and then it finds a worm or a grasshopper to eat, but it's doubtful. The bird simply wouldn't know what to do with an insect.

Then there's the 'organic' free-range chicken. These birds eat organic wheat or corn, but are otherwise no different to the base chicken or the non-organic free-range variety. Better, but only slightly.

And just for a bit of fun … what colour's a chicken? I asked my children this question and they answered 'white'. Well, for a long time when I was growing up, chickens were yellow. The phrase 'to be chicken', or a coward, came from the meaning 'to be yellow'. But which came first, the chicken, or the egg? I think 'being chicken' came first, suggesting our first reaction is to run from danger - hence the expression 'being yellow' ('yeller' if you're American). But chickens today are white, and that's for two reasons; their poor diet, and because they're dipped in chlorine prior to being delivered to you. The chlorine decreases the risk of salmonella infection (food poisoning). Another word for chlorine is bleach, so the chicken is 'bleached' white. I mean I don't want salmonella, but I really prefer unchlorinated chicken as well.

If I can get hold of one, I'll buy an organic free-range, pastured chicken. The breeds don't change a great deal, nor does the feed, but the bird probably spends far more time outside, therefore it obtains more vitamin D. The reason this chicken is labelled as 'organic', is because the grain it eats is organic grain. It's still not the bird's natural diet, but better than most. Let's score this chicken a 5, compared to the base value of 1.

Another good question…if a chicken's natural diet consists of grasshoppers and worms, why wouldn't it eat them, instead of the grain it's fed? Answer: for many reasons, but the main one being that these chickens are housed between 3000 or 10,000 per hectare. There simply aren't enough worms to go round. And here's another: If you were to put children in a room full of lollies and sausages, which food would they eat? Yes, the lollies of course. They have loads of calories, are easy to chew, and they taste great. Grain's like that too; instant calories, no hassle, so naturally the chicken eats the grain first. No need for chasing, catching, digging, so no energy wasted and it tastes good.

When I can get them, I buy naturally raised, old breed chickens that spend most of their life outdoors eating grasshoppers and worms. They're not fed unnatural diets of grain. There's a guy in Victoria that breeds these chickens. The birds are 200 days old when their lives end, as opposed to 60 days for the base chicken variety. The meat on my 'super chicken' is beautiful…it tastes nutritious and satisfying. The naturally raised, old breed chickens weigh around 4kg and cost $100 each. They're mostly purchased by high-end restaurants and the farmer doesn't have any problem selling them.

If you eat two organic free-range chickens a month, you'll pay around $40 for 4kg of chicken. That would equate to a total of eight servings for a family of four (x 2 meals). The naturally raised, old breed chickens provide around 12 servings, and it's far more nutritious. If you're eating the base chicken, you'll likely also need a vitamin supplement. They will cost you around $10 to make up for what you're missing out on in your regular chicken, but not much more in the scheme of things. Taking all into account, I assume my super chicken will still cost you more, but not much. I can assure you, try it once and you'll be hooked. They're not easy to find, but well worth the effort when you do. I score my super chicken a 10, but then again, I'm biased.

It's understandable to try and get more calories for your money. For humans, calories have been our primary pursuit for thousands of years. Obtaining calories today is no longer a problem, but the quality of them certainly is. I'd never presume to judge you for buying lesser quality food. I did the same myself for many years, and still do when I can't source those lovely chickens I like. I guess my message is: Live life fully and get what you can out of it. Just don't forget that quality food should be your priority. Everything else becomes cheaper and more satisfying when you do.

I often observe people who are obese and wonder about them. I am currently overweight at 220lb (100kg) and 6ft tall...would much prefer to be around 190lb, which is normal for me. No one intentionally becomes overweight. Everyone would like to be beautiful and thin. So why aren't they? I believe the answer is quite simple. Forget what anyone tells you about balanced diets, exercise and moderation. That rarely seems to work. Concentrate on consuming top quality, natural foods. If you go for quality over quantity, I believe you'll achieve your goals.

It's not easy - take baby steps and in the end you'll be rewarded. Your diet is far more important than gym sessions, Netflix, your next holiday, or some great 4WD adventure. The quality of food you eat should absolutely be the number one goal of your existence for optimal mental and physical health.

Now I'm going to throw the vegans and veggos a bone here. At least they have the perception of good health at the core of their being. They aren't executing their choices in the correct way it, but at least they're trying. If you're a regular person like me and love your meat, get the best stuff that your money can buy...you will be rewarded. It may appear more expensive, but that's just a perception, not reality. Your health will improve, you'll require fewer supplements and medicines, so you might just find that consuming quality food is cheaper in the long run.

Superfoods

This is an area I've discussed with a few people and it's a concept really, not a rule. If you require a substance; plant, medicine, herb, or vitamin, that's produced high up in the Himalayas, or from a pristine mountain stream in Peru or Kazakhstan to make your diet complete, or fix your ailment, then it sounds like an unsustainable model to me. The key to your health and mental wellbeing shouldn't be far from where you live. Make it yourself, or source it from someone who doesn't only have 'profit' in mind. Go for good, down-to-earth natural foods that have stood the test of time.

My Prescription of Natural Foods

Have one meal a week, or one meal a day (if possible) of pure, natural, unadulterated food. This is much harder than you may think, but certainly achievable. My perfect meal is roast lamb with all the trimmings - those lambs aren't crazy enough to eat grain. They feed on their mother's milk and she doesn't eat grain either...only grass. Sheep are basically your processing factory, where sunshine is converted into products you can digest. Then you have to cook it of course. Personally, I like meat cooked through so there's no blood, but you can cook it however you want to. If you live in the USA or some other joint where you can't get lamb, have beef instead, but make sure it's grass-fed beef. Again, there's science behind this.

If you're a vegetarian, I feel sorry for you, but you could use fish if you have to. It must be fish caught in the wild, not farmed fish.

If you're a vegan, then I doubt you're reading this book anyway, so it doesn't matter that much. 'Come back to the other side' is my only advice. It may be okay to be a vegan for six days of the week (though I doubt it), but one day a week gorging on meat or fish will probably help you. Again, I digress.

So roast lamb with gravy, made from the fat of the lamb, and roasted vegetables is my prescription. One meal will not cure your Depression, but it will make you feel better. If you did this for a week, without drinking poison like diet sodas and sugar substitutes, or eating take-away food (most of it), I reckon you'd make big progress. Again, if you die of cholesterol poisoning after eating the meal I've recommended then call me and I'll send a wreath.

SPOOKY STORY

- <u>VEGETABLES WERE ONLY INVENTED YESTERDAY!</u> -

Ah…that got your attention! I'm talking about the 'metaphorical' yesterday, like in the past five hundred years.

This is the theory I propose…

Imagine yourself say five hundred years ago. When you were hungry, you'd trap a deer or rabbit, kill a cow, or catch a fish. If those options weren't available to you during midwinter, a drought, or some other catastrophe, then you had to go looking for some other source of calories. So what about fruit or vegetables? Good thinking…but there aren't any. In winter when the ground's covered with snow, the only thing growing are trees, and you can't eat them. So your only choice would be to dig for root vegetables that grow underground; carrots, turnips, beetroot, radish, or cassava.

Going back five hundred years, there weren't any potatoes, unless you were American. If there were any lettuces or zucchinis (though zucchinis have only existed for two hundred years) on the surface, they would have already been devoured by bunny rabbits, cows, deer, moose, and rats. These animals aren't good at digging so they eat the surface plants first. There are some exceptions to this rule; cabbage and broccoli for example. Bunnies don't eat them because these vegetables taste bitter and contain indigestible chemicals like oxalic acid. We need to cook or ferment cabbage before we eat it, so that it doesn't irritate the gut. I mean you'd obviously eat it if you had nothing else, but your first choice would always be meat or fish. So, surface vegetables were rare five hundred years ago. I'm not saying they weren't eaten, just a 'last option', and that's if they were even available at all.

Other plant-based foods were occasionally available like bananas, mangoes, oranges and apples. You just had to be lucky enough to pick them before the birds, bats, grasshoppers and fruit flies got to them. Plants were never designed to feed humans. Their purpose is to nourish the seeds of the fruit and vegetables. This allows the maximum chance for their survival. They can then create a new bush, tree, or plant, to keep the species going.

Hey, don't get me wrong...I love my fresh fruit and veggies. They're obviously not poison. But if you suffer from Depression, I'd encourage against being vegetarian or vegan, just for a while anyway. It's far less 'natural' than you'd think it is. Solve your Depression problem now and save the planet later. Save yourself first. Besides, I'm not convinced that you're saving the earth by eating plant foods (that's an argument for another book, and probably by someone smarter than me).

Anything that's fat reduced, salt reduced, supplemented with vitamins or iron is suspect. Eat as fresh and as natural as your budget will allow.

CHAPTER 17

Genetics

It's difficult to reveal within a few pages, what I've learned about genes in a digestible way. The main thing in relation to Depression is that your genes, and your DNA, are far less important than you are led to believe.

We're all pretty much the same; far more 'similar' than we are 'different' is the key here.

Genes are far less important than you think

Humans possess around 20,000 genes. Bananas have 30,000. Does this make humans more, or less complex, than a banana? Well genetically speaking, bananas are 50% more complex, but I'd back my son's football team against the world's best banana team any time.

Here's another one: Humans in fact have between 20,000 and 25,000 genes. So, if we assume the middle is around 22,500, then the variation is about 11%, plus or minus. We're told that chimpanzees share about 96% of human genes. So chances are you have more genetically in common with a chimp in Africa, than you do with your next-door neighbour or spouse.

Look, that's just playing with pure numbers, not biology. But numbers are important too.

The most genetically complex animal found in the world thus far, is a tiny little water flea (Daphnia), and it has 31,000 genes.

How about this then? In your gut (mostly), but on your skin, in your appendix and mouth, are trillions of bacteria (about 100 trillion). There are a thousand species of bacteria on any average person. Each species of bacteria contain about 3000 genes. So, your bacteria contain around three million genes, or 99.4% of genes in your body are bacterial genes, not human genes. They ebb and flow as species are replaced by other species. You'll destroy more genes with a single dose of antibiotics than almost any other method. Destroying plenty of genes is not something I'd do lightly...but you know, I'm not against antibiotics (when required).

Your genes are important to the way you look, walk, your hair colour, and eye colour. As far as internal plumbing and chemistry are concerned, we're all pretty much the same. Chemistry in particular is a law, not a theory. Chemical reactions in one person are the same as in another. The way that chemistry reacts with your genes may vary, but not by much. There are also genes that are turned on and off, do different things at different times, or become activated or deactivated (generally due to environmental factors). This is why I personally think that genetics have far less to do with an illness like Depression than we're led to believe.

If you share a disease like Diabetes, Depression or Gout with one of your close relatives, it probably has a lot more to do with shared environmental factors than it does to do with shared genes. It may have more to do with shared bacteria, but we just don't know enough about those things yet.

There is one gene that I know a little about, not much, but it's worth telling the story. I call it the COMT gene defect. I have it, as previously mentioned, but it's not really a 'defect' because around 40% of the population have it. In practical terms, a person with the COMT defect has trouble processing B vitamins. At least that's what it appears on the surface. But they're really battling with the processing of 'synthetic' B vitamins; the type sold in pill form. And they didn't exist fifty years ago. It's hardly a defect, or a weakness. As I said in the vitamin chapter, get your vitamins from real food, the way nature intended, and you won't have a problem.

In Short on Genes

I encourage you not to fall for the story that you have Depression because of your genes, regardless of 'evidence' that it's in your family. It just isn't mathematically possible. If you have, or ever had genes that caused Depression, evolution would have worked you out 100,000 years ago, and you simply wouldn't be here today. The 'excuse' that it's in your genes just gives you less motivation to do something about it. It may well be in your family, but that will have much more to do with your shared environment, rather than your physical makeup.

CHAPTER 18

Data Manipulation

I'll tell you how easy it is to manipulate data to tell a story that you want heard.

I was listening to an officer from Queensland Police on ABC radio a few months ago. He was talking about road fatalities and how to reduce the numbers; a noble cause no doubt. He discussed the importance of wearing seatbelts and wheeled out a statistic that went like this...

Around 25% of all road fatalities occur when the person is not wearing a seat belt. So the message is: 'Seat Belts Save Lives', you should wear one. I'm fully in acceptance of that argument.

But then I started toying with the numbers in my head. If 25% of all fatalities occur to those <u>not</u> wearing a seat belt, then 75% of deaths happen to people who <u>are</u> wearing seatbelts. Let's say the numbers are 200 road deaths per year in Queensland, which is about right. That means fifty people die each year on our roads that are not wearing a seatbelt. In turn, the remaining 150 deaths occur to people who <u>are</u> wearing a seat belt. You 'could' draw the conclusion that you're three times more likely to die if you wear a seatbelt. Obviously that's the wrong conclusion, but it goes to show how simple data manipulation is...even I can do it.

Pharmaceutical companies design tests, before they even start the test, to ensure the best chance of proving what they want to prove.

It's natural to want a positive outcome. I don't know if it's particularly scientific, but it's definitely commercial. Anyway, if the tests start showing adverse effects, they abandon the trials part way through, and usually don't publish the data. If the adverse effects aren't too awful, they'll redesign the trial to change things like location, the participants, the reporting period, even the dosage. The next time they run the trial, their chances of a positive outcome improve. It doesn't always work out. By the time they've reached clinical trials though, they've already invested a lot of money, so they really need to be successful.

Gardasil is the HPV (Human Papillomavirus Vaccine) vaccine. When the early pre-trials were carried out in Denmark, it should have been possible for the Guinea pigs/paid volunteers to report any adverse effects within say 6 months, or even one month after the trial inoculation. Those effects also should have been recorded, regardless of whether it could be attributed to the vaccine or not. I mean if there were suddenly a spate of car accidents, broken legs, or an outbreak of flu in the participants, which was out of step with the general population, then it should be noted, regardless of attributing to the drug or not. Instead, in the pre-trials, the reporting period was restricted to fourteen days, and proof that the adverse effect was related to the vaccine was required, otherwise it wasn't reported.

I'm not suggesting for one minute that Gardasil is unsafe. You'll have to make your own decision about that. You should also weigh up exactly 'what' you're protecting yourself/your child from, and whether the risks are worth it. It goes back to a statement I made earlier in the book. 'You never get something for nothing', Newtons Law, for every action there is an equal and opposite reaction. It's possible that Gardasil will turn out to be very beneficial. We may know the answer to that in thirty years, but we don't know it yet. I mean it's not like mumps, measles, rubella, or polio. HPV is a disease which is extremely unlikely to kill or harm you for many years into the future.

Vaccinations

I'm not an anti vaxxer, but mass vaccinations have only been around for forty years or so. We know that vaccinations save people from Mumps, Rubella and Measles for example. I don't know how I managed it, but I had all of those diseases as a child, and somehow, I survived. I also had chicken pox and the flu. I wasn't a sickly kid, pretty average as far as my health was concerned.

I used to give some advice to people, or offer a saying that went like this...if you want to have good health and live a long life...you'd better be born before 1970. That year reference is just arbitrary; think I picked it purely because it was around then that our food supply started to be compromised. Mass immunisations started growing in popularity, with antibiotics being the first line of treatment. Vitamins in pill form took off too.

There's a vaccination that's popular today called MMR. It's the Measles, Mumps and Rubella (Rubella in English means German measles). Apparently, all of these diseases are serious. That may be the case. If you live in the real world and contract all three diseases at once, you die. It would be just like having Typhoid, Cholera, and Malaria all at the same time, I reckon you'd die. Anyway, apparently you can inject a tiny bit of each disease into a child (all at once) and they will develop antibodies. Nothing else will happen. So we start injecting it into developing babies. We don't do this after their immune system is fully developed. Instead, we administer the injection well before maturity, which naturally occurs between 2 to 3 years of age. If you think about it a bit, you'll realise that it's more of an organisational reason, rather than a medical one. The average length of time that a mother nurses her baby is around 18 months to two years. Her average time between births is probably around 2.5 years. So if the child is immunised at say 12 to 18 months, there's a lot less organisation required, because the mother has her full attention on that child. It has nothing to do with any medical reason. And if you stick them all in one vaccination, you only have to visit the doctor once, instead of three times.

Now people assume there must be solid medical research behind vaccinating 12-month-old babies with three serious diseases at the same time. It must be safe, right? I don't know if quality research has been conducted, but I doubt it.

The standard for scientific testing is called a double-blind placebo-controlled test. I wonder how many mothers would offer up their baby to participate in the testing of a new drug/vaccination? For thorough testing, the baby would have to be followed for years, not months, to determine any long-term effects. You also need a second group of babies that don't have the injection (for comparison), and follow them for years too. The two groups then have to be compared on many different measures. I'm suggesting there's a possibility that this type of testing has never been carried out on children this young, or followed for years. Therefore it hasn't been placebo controlled. If I happen to be wrong, I stand corrected. I mean, imagine the conversation in the doctor's office:

> "Excuse me Susan, would you like your one-year-old to participate in the study of a new vaccination that combines three deadly viruses all at once? We've tried it in rats, monkeys, and Pakistani children, and that seemed to work … hardly any of them died. The only downside is that we can't tell you whether your child received the real vaccine, or the placebo, for about five years."

> "Sure, why not, just pump whatever you like into little Johnny. I'm sure he'll be fine. Do I get paid?"

It just seems implausible, that's all.

In relation to MMR in particular, just to let you know…in the EU, MMR vaccines are routinely separated into single vaccines. Maybe they're smarter than us, I don't know.

By the way, all of my children are 'more or less' fully immunised, except for the Gardasil vaccine (a recent Australian invention). Because my wife is so brilliant and has a PhD in Microbiology (you know, the study of tiny living things), our children were immunised at the last possible moment, allowing their small bodies time to develop a stronger immune system. As most of you would know, there's a vast difference between a baby at 12 months old and one at 2-3 years of age. We received an awful lot of pressure from the government to have these immunisations earlier. They even threatened to cut off our child support payments... oh no... how would we survive without those monthly cheques for zero dollars?

An interesting article below:

> *"Trials of HPV vaccine may have overestimated its efficacy, study finds...*
>
> *The efficacy of human papillomavirus (HPV) vaccines as a preventative for cervical cancer may have been overestimated in trials, a review in the Journal of the Royal Society of Medicine has concluded (21 January 2020)."*
>
> (Web source: https://www.pharmaceutical-journal.com/news-and-analysis/research-briefing/trials-of-hpv-vaccine-may-have-overestimated-its-efficacy-study-finds/20207648.article?firstPass=false)

Basically the trials were not followed up for long enough. Mostly just 6 years, but cervical cancer takes decades to develop. Then there was the fact that all the trial participants were around 18 years old. The (girls) that were being vaccinated were to be 9-13 years old. I don't know about other countries, but in Australia we are now giving it to 10 year old boys, how clever are we?"

The point is that vaccinations have been documented for efficacy and safety, but have they been evaluated for really young kids? All vaccinations aren't the same - what works for one virus may not work on another. Something that works for bacteria (Tetanus) may not work for viruses. There's a massive case on both sides of the argument regarding vaccinations. Even the common cold is a virus, and we still don't have a vaccination for it. The flu virus vaccine is available, but its only 60% successful. Tossing a coin is a good method too, it's about 50% efficient. Is there a downside to the flu vaccination? You bet … sometimes it gives you the flu. All I'm saying is that when it comes to your health, don't believe everything you read or hear, even when it becomes 'common knowledge'.

Let's just say that vaccines are another 'little thing' that has changed in the world, and again, we really have no long-term epidemiological placebo-controlled studies to validate these experiments.

When I was a boy it was common for overseas travellers to be vaccinated for Typhoid, Cholera, and Yellow Fever. It seriously bothered me because I'd watch my parents receive them, knowing the injections hurt, then they'd usually be quite ill for a few days afterward. Back then I didn't care for travelling overseas, I preferred to stay at home and not get jabbed. All adults seemed to do it willingly though, and you certainly could die from any one of these diseases in the unlikely event that you contracted it. Question is … why didn't they just stick all of those diseases together in one shot? I'll tell you why: because it might kill you.

Anyway, now that we're so much smarter, we've worked out how to make these vaccinations more acceptable to our bodies. We can put three, allegedly deadly diseases together in the one vaccine, and give it to a one-year old child. Yeah, that's super clever. Does anyone ever ask; "But should we? Is there the chance of any undesirable consequences?" I know a few people who want their children to contract some of these diseases, like Chicken Pox for example. Once your kids get it, it seems to strengthen and mature them, then it's over and done with basically for life. There's even such a thing as 'Chicken Pox Parties'. The host is an infected kid who invites all the other kids to make sure they get it too. Just so you know, these people aren't crazy, they're everyday people like you and me. I've seen it in my own children; after a fever they seem to awaken with newfound maturity.

The Chicken Pox vaccine was introduced en masse in the USA in 1995. That was only twenty-five years ago. Therefore it's not possible to conclude long-term epidemiological studies. There are plenty of people who point to the success of the Polio vaccine. Fair enough, but that doesn't mean exactly the same mechanism is at play for all other viruses or diseases. And it doesn't mean you can put three viruses in the one vaccination safely either. Anyway, I digress as usual. What I'm saying is that when it comes to your health, it's worth taking some time and responsibility for yourself. Think about these things and do some research. Blind faith isn't good enough. Accessing information is easy today, so take some responsibility for your health and use the internet to your benefit.

'Merck', a giant, German Pharmaceutical company (or their Australian Subsidiary), even published their own 'Australasian Journal of Bone and Joint Medicine'. On the surface it appeared to be an independent medical journal but was it in fact, primarily to help sell Merck products like Fosamax and Vioxx? Note: They can't sue me for saying this because it has already been proven in court.

Vioxx has been withdrawn from the market due to serious side effects and Fosamax is facing millions in pending and finalised lawsuits, due to possible, serious side effects.

Maybe I'm an idealist, I don't know. What I do find, even with my own friends, is that it's quite difficult to see cause and effect. There are just so many competing factors today, so many variables in all our lives, that it's hard to know what does what.

Now here's a good story, one of my favourites about Warren and Marshall, two Australian research scientists who unexpectedly and virtually accidentally discovered that stomach ulcers were caused by a bacterium called Helicobacter Pylori (HP) and that the ulcers could be cured with antibiotics. The discovery was made in 1985. It took <u>twenty</u>

<u>years later</u> for that therapy to hit the market and now 95% of stomach ulcers are cured this way. Warren and Marshall won the Nobel Prize for their work in 2005. Maybe not everything I said above is completely accurate, but it's close enough. The question is: Why did it take so long for their ulcer cure to hit the market, or become accepted? I'm very willing to speculate here. Gastroenterologists, (doctors who treat ulcers) just didn't want to know about it, nor did the drug companies. Ulcer medication was a very lucrative business, so they hardly wanted to run around curing everyone. Or it could be that once the patent on the ulcer drugs ran out (usually 21 years), there'd be little profit left, so interest in that income stream reduced.

Now I'm not a conspiracy theorist, even if I sound like one. I prefer to think of myself as a realist, so I'm coining a new phrase...I'm an observationist.

In terms of conspiracies, maybe there are a few out there. I'm sure there are. What's more important is that it's perfectly natural for human beings to want to protect their turf, make money, and repeat that as often as possible.

I used to have statistics (that I lost) on the most profitable companies worldwide, before the tech giants took over. Sorry, I can't find it. What I did find though was that Pharmaceutical companies feature highly amongst the group. Pfizer for example, a year or so ago, yielded a staggering 43% profit. Maybe drug companies made the list by curing the world's health problems...a fair enough assumption. What I'm saying is that these guys are seriously good at making money. So perhaps, every now and then, the data gets skewed in their favour.

Even in the great 'Framingham Study' that I mentioned previously, data can often be 'suppressed' or manipulated. For example, it was found in the late 1960s that there was no correlation between cholesterol and dietary saturated fat intake. There was also no connection between cholesterol and heart disease. And: *"Men in the same physical activity class tend to have higher serum cholesterol levels at lower caloric intake. This finding is contrary to expectation."*

So instead of publishing these findings in a well-known medical journal, which would have been easy, the information was more or less buried where it would be hard to find. It was just so contrary to what they expected to find and the message they wanted known.

The Depression industry is a huge behemoth. There are doctors, counsellors, and all sorts of people dedicated, and genuinely interested in helping you become well, but it's a never-ending struggle.

What if? What if I'm right, and all you need to do is change your diet and fix your gut bacteria? Hey, it's a lot cheaper than all that other stuff, less time consuming, and your only risk is the cost of a better piece of steak, properly cooked food, and a trip to the beach for your sunshine... maybe a bottle of probiotics for a month or two as well. Keep seeing your counsellor or psychiatrist by all means, just add in a couple of my suggestions too and see what happens.

So, in terms of Depression I suggest this: If you have it, the model that you're using doesn't work for some reason. You'll have to run some new experiments. Don't necessarily believe all the medical data and don't necessarily believe me. You can only assume that your doctor, counsellor, and I, have your best interests at heart. The problem here is, we're human too, so we can also be mislead by data. And the medics have their own associations whom they're more or less compelled to adhere to.

My own doctor admits that there's no way known for him to keep up with the Tsunami of new data he's supposed to remain abreast of. That's another form of data manipulation... just flood the market with data, so no one knows which way to turn.

Data is, in itself, a modern invention. Before it, we only had stories and anecdotes. That being said, they're important; sometimes more important than data.

I read a lovely story in *Spectator Magazine,* October 2018.

It was about the Babylonians (Iraqis) and how they solved their health problems thousands of years ago. The afflicted person would hang out in the town square during the day. Any passers-by were obliged (by law) to ask them the nature of their illness. The passer-by would then have to offer advice, if they could, regrading anyone they knew with a similar problem. That way most of the illnesses were solved, or cured. There's a good example of stories and anecdotes and as doctors' magazines have observed; 'as everyday experience and doctors' advice columns testify, who does not adore talking about their own ailments and advising others on what has worked for them?'"

Don't overrate data, and don't underrate stories.

PS.

There's a common drug called Lipitor. It's used for treating high cholesterol. I took it for a short while, but I had strong side effects; very sore muscles. According to the official literature, muscle soreness occurs in about 2/1000 patients (0.002). I have conducted my own survey of friends, family, and acquaintances that take, or have taken Lipitor. My research tells me that side effects occur in 80% of the group I surveyed. To be fair, I'm talking about less than twenty people. Maybe my data collection wasn't up to scratch. There just seems to be a big difference between my stats, 800/1000 compared to the official stats of 2/1000.

The original tests on cholesterol were conducted around a hundred years ago in Russia. Cholesterol was fed to a bunch of rabbits and they developed arterial blockages and other health problems like atherosclerosis. Rabbits are vegetarians and don't normally consume cholesterol. No wonder they had trouble digesting it. Those tests are still one of the foundations we use today for the cholesterol/saturated fat/heart health hypothesis. That theory has certainly sold a lot of drugs.

The vast majority of drugs have their roots in animal trials. I'm all for it (sorry rats and bunnies). You just have to be careful with this method. The closest animal to our own system is probably the dog. Everyone loves dogs, which is why they're not commonly used in animal trials. They also live too long and eat a lot. The point is, you can't take a vegetarian animal like a rat or a bunny, and conduct dietary trials, thinking you have a solution. It's just a guess, at best. Once you get into the data gathering business, it's so easy to manipulate data in your favour. You should be careful of data, whether you're a layman like me, or a trained professional. Do your best to make sure you're not being lied to... it's a common occurrence.

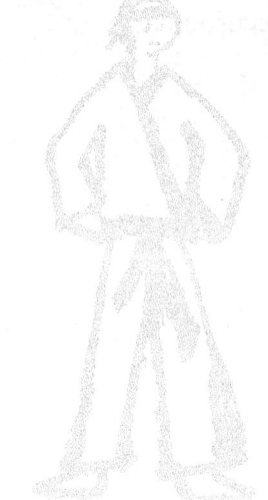

CHAPTER 19

Politics in Medicine

What, there's politics in medicine? Of course there is. There's politics in science, in your soccer team, your household, and even in your head. You can say that you have no interest in politics, but if you're human, and I suspect you are, then you're involved in a political game all the time. You could call it hierarchy if you wanted to, but there's a constant competition of ideas, protocols, acceptance, rejection, and prioritising going on all the time. That's basically politics, but I digress as usual.

The subject here is 'politics in medicine', and it affects how easily you'll cure your Depression. Because I'm not a doctor, I don't have to comply with their politics, the AMA, or any other professional body for that matter, but they do. This gives me an edge to some extent.

When it comes to your overall health and wellbeing, your doctor has all sorts of competing interests to comply with.

When I talk about the importance of sunshine, or salt, or bacteria, I can do that, but if I were an affiliated doctor, I certainly couldn't. I'm bound by my own organisation, which is in turn bound by all sorts of competing interests.

Let's take sunshine as an example.

The American Society of Dermatologists suggests that the amount of sunshine you can safely consume is zero. The Dermatologists are concerned about your skin and skin cancer. Skin cancer is a huge problem, there's no doubt, but almost all skin cancers are of the non-fatal kind. The fatal type is called Melanoma.

Melanoma seems not exclusively affected by sun exposure. For example, many melanomas are found under people's feet or on top of their head (which is normally covered with hair). And to tell you the truth, if any person deserves to have skin cancer, it's me. When I was a kid, I spent endless time in the sun, without much protection. My nose would peel so many times that it'd bleed. My mother tried to get me to cover up, but it didn't work too well. I've had some minor skin cancers on my chest and arms, but if any area 'deserved' a skin cancer, it would be my nose, ears, or face. In fact, my nickname at school was 'Bacon'. Not because I was fat or liked pork, but because I'd go to school on a Monday after a weekend at the beach, thin, red, and fried. Again, I digress.

So even if a doctor was to read my book, witness first-hand how getting more sunshine effects people's positive mental health, conduct experiments on his own family, or research and find evidence confirming the hypothesis, he'd be going way out on a limb if he told you to get more sun exposure.

The same goes for salt. The Heart Foundation and cardiologists would have your doctor's head if they knew he was recommending more salt consumption. It's particularly hard for general practitioners; slightly easier for specialists, but they too have to be careful. Then there's the financial aspect of it all. It isn't good for psychiatrists to be recommending more salt, sunshine, clean water, and grass-fed meat either. Not only would they be in trouble with their professional body, they'd also get a slap on the wrist from drug companies.

They'd prefer to sell you a drug, and if all their patients recover, they destroy their own business model. I'm not suggesting that your doctor or psychiatrist doesn't want you to get better, they certainly do, but their hands are tied to some extent by professional organisations, and their insurers.

Do you recall the story of Warren and Marshall in the last chapter? They're the doctors who basically cured ulcers. The gastro guys didn't want to know. It killed their business model and the drug companies' profits. That's politics in medicine at its very best ... and not just politics, it's also human nature. Protect your turf, make money, and protect your ass. I'm not being cynical, seriously. It's just the nature of the world. We all do it and we're all guilty of it, even me, I'm sure.

Pharmaceutical companies are amongst the most profitable companies in the world. These guys are seriously smart bastards. They know every way to manipulate data, governments, systems, and people. Possibly the most useful and safest synthetic drug to ever hit the market was Aspirin, developed by Bayer in Munich. All their competitors were jealous and wanted to put their own 'far less useful' drugs on the market. These rival companies dredged the research to find something, anything, to discredit Aspirin, so they could sell useless products like paracetamol. Aspirin was demonised by a rare condition called Raynaud's Syndrome. There's very flimsy evidence that Aspirin causes this condition, but there was just enough to aid in Aspirin's demise. That made way for new profits, generated by new painkillers that were much less effective.

Cod liver oil and Aspirin are some of the best drugs/supplements to ever hit the market. So what the drug companies want to ensure is that no one recovers too quickly or cheaply, because it isn't a great business model. Saturated fat, salt, and sunshine were demonised in similar ways, leading to a great financial model for all sorts of businesses.

Dexibuprofen

Following on with anti-inflammatory drugs, and politics in medicine ...

I was in Austria six months ago, beautiful country, but there was too much snow. I experienced an incredible toothache: a cracked tooth underneath a filling. Because we were travelling, I had limited access to painkillers and dentists. Red wine became my painkiller, which worked reasonably well.

One Saturday night the pain got really bad. I asked my wife to accompany me to the hospital for some pain relief (her German is way better than mine). I ended up with a $10 prescription for Dexibuprofen. It's similar to Ibuprofen, which I thought would be basically useless. Well it worked, and it worked fast. So I did a bit of research on it. This will be slightly challenging for many readers, but give it a go.

Ibuprofen is made up of two isomers. It's very much like table sugar, which also contains two isomers. This means there are two molecules with the same chemical formula, but they're a different shape. Some call it 'mirror images' of one another, which is close enough. With sugar (sucrose) the isomers are called fructose and glucose. Fructose is sweet and turns to fat in your system. Glucose is energy, though not really sweet. With Ibuprofen, the two isomers are named 'R' and 'S'. The 'S' isomer is the painkiller. The 'R' isomer is just along for the ride. A bit like sugar... glucose is energy, fructose is sort of useless. In Ibuprofen the 'R' isomer does nothing for your pain. Worse than that, the 'R' isomer gets in the way of the 'S' isomer. So the question is, why don't we just use the 'S' isomer for pain relief when it's obviously possible to separate the two?

Well here are some suggestions. There are costs associated with the purification process, so pharmaceutical companies prefer not to do it. But the price is negligible, so that's not enough of an answer. When you take regular Ibuprofen, you'll need at least double the amount to solve your pain. So the drug companies sell two tablets instead of one. This almost doubles sales and profits, right? Then there's the therapeutic effect. They can't just go around solving all problems, or their sales would plummet. Even with strong tooth pain, I reduced the Dexibuprofen dose down to ½ a tablet, twice a day. I was attempting to save on tablets because they were so helpful. If I was taking normal Ibuprofen, the dose would be two tablets, four times a day…and the pain relief wouldn't be near as good. Now because it's almost exactly the same drug, it's unlikely that its addictive, or that the side effects are less tolerated. The only difference is that the 'S' isomer (Dexibuprofen) is more effective. But you can't just run around selling more effective drugs, as you know, that would destroy your business model. I've hunted for Dexibuprofen in Australia and overseas. It's extremely hard to come by, and then usually only by prescription, whereas the much less useful Ibuprofen is sold in supermarkets.

That's why Aspirin was demonised: because it's so effective. The Americans stole it from the Germans, after the war. The spoils of war, as they say. In 1945 or thereabouts, Aspirin was the world's number one drug and it was very effective. Not just for pain relief, but it did many other things as well, like thinning the blood, which is great if your blood happens to be too thick, or your blood pressure's too high. It's quite effective for stroke prevention. I mean there are side effects as with every drug, but they're mild. Even better than Aspirin is willow bark. Aspirin is a synthetic version of willow bark, but that's another argument. If you use Aspirin for blood thinning and stroke prevention, it probably costs around 10c a day or less. Now there's another drug for blood thinning that has been in use for some years now: Warfarin. It costs around $3 a day when you include the cost of the drug itself, and the testing that goes along with it. Warfarin has way more side effects, so why not just use Aspirin? Well many people do, but if you're a drug company, it's far more fun to produce an expensive drug with greater side effects, especially if you can get someone to pay for it.

So what does this have to do with Depression? Well, it's sort of a warning that you need to do some research on the drugs you're taking, any drugs, and not just blindly accept the word of health professionals and drug companies. Look for the mechanism they're trying to treat, and find out why. Very often, there's an angle you could be missing. Read the literature on the drug you're prescribed, and don't believe its claims of how 'rare' certain side effects are. The reporting of adverse effects just isn't good enough for anyone to know. Look at the user forums on the internet too. There's a lot of honesty out there, and loads of people wanting to tell their stories.

I'm quite sure I'll receive a bit of push-back over this book. There are plenty of people hoping that I'm not right. Those who are far cleverer and more highly trained than I, count on the fact that I'm wrong...their very livelihoods depend on it.

The World is Round

I'm not quite old enough to remember when the world was flat, but I've heard it said. Galileo lost his life proving that the sun, not the earth, was the centre of the solar system. He was right, but they killed him anyway. Until Australia was discovered, there was no such thing as a black swan either. It was merely a fairy tale. Some people still don't believe that man landed on the moon. I believe, but I have no proof. Even proof can be over, or under-rated.

I would really rather you perform a few short term, low risk experiments, like taking probiotics, upping your salt, getting more sunshine, and filtering your water. It's just easier than buying into all the politics of health recommendations.

Depression is primarily caused by antibiotic use. Perhaps it can be alleviated by sun, salt, and probiotics. Who's to say this isn't true...and what do you have to lose by testing my theory?

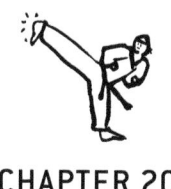

CHAPTER 20

Double Blinded Placebo Controlled Studies

If you're not familiar with DBPCS (Double Blinded Placebo Controlled Studies), this is the 'Gold Standard' for testing drugs. For example:

You have two groups with an ailment like Depression. One group is given a drug, while the other group is given a placebo (a salt or sugar tablet for example). The people who administer the drugs don't know which group is receiving which. That's the double-blind bit. The Guinea pigs don't know, and neither do the doctors. There's a weird thing known as the 'placebo effect' whereby some 30% of the group become well, as do a portion of the group receiving the drug. I'd need to write another book to get into that subject, but I'm digressing again. Strangely, I often hear from doctors, patients, and medical people that these DBPCS studies are the only type they'll accept. It's understandable I suppose.

Thing is, these same people (us), accept so many things in life without any testing at all. Even if tests actually indicate harm, we still accept them. I'll give you an example: Driving a car. Road accidents kill people every day. Do we stop driving our cars? Of course not, because we believe the risks are outweighed by the benefits. And that's a rational decision...plenty of benefits, and the associated risks are very low. I mentioned earlier in the book how numerous changes, along with plenty of experiments we run on a daily basis, show no evidence of being beneficial to our health. Hot water showers, underarm deodorant, flying in planes, the use of mobile phones, consumption of vegetable oils, vitamin tablets etc, just to name a few. All we do know is that we don't tend to die from doing these things, overnight anyway. The risks seem manageable. Now I'm not for one second suggesting you try anything crazy like taking a synthetic drug that hasn't been rigorously tested. I'm suggesting you test a series of low-risk experiments, like getting more sunshine, salt, good water, and probiotics.

It has been suggested to me that I conduct tests based on my theories in relation to Depression; you know, a Double blinded Placebo controlled study. But that would take years and the results would be rejected for various reasons. Besides, the cost alone would be enormous. Here are just some of the reasons for rejection: sample sizes would be too small, so they're unrepresentative, and because 30% of the people in the placebo group would become well. There are so many reasons to reject findings. For example, the sunshine in Queensland is very different to New York. And the list would go on. The reason that pharmaceutical companies love the DBPCS is… 1: They're very wealthy and profitable, so this forms a barrier to almost everyone who isn't, which is most of us. 2: Sunshine, salt, and water aren't patentable, so there's no interest in conducting a study if you don't 'own the results. 3: There's no money in it if it's successful.

The main reason that the Malaria problem hasn't been solved, in my opinion, is that Malaria is only really an issue in poor countries today. There's no money in solving problems in poor countries, so why do it? I saw some figures the other day where the USA sucks in around half of the world's expenditure on pharmaceuticals. They're only 4% of the world's population and relatively speaking, also close to the world's healthiest population. The pharmaceutical industry doesn't have much time for cures either; there isn't enough money in it. Management programs are far more profitable. So it's basically a case of 'take this pill daily for the rest of your life and your problem will be managed'. The industry then receives an income stream for life.

I've also toyed with this idea. Let's say you wanted to find out if hot water is good or bad for your skin. How do you even conduct a DBPCS on this subject? It's impossible, because those who receive the hot water will know they're receiving it. I mean you could do a population-sized study and plot hot water usage against longevity, and as hard as it might be, you would end up with a result. But does it mean anything?

This is basically another example of politics in medicine. Please don't let me sell you the idea that our world is an evil place, or not to trust doctors or pharmaceutical companies. I'm well open to the idea that their main aim is your health and wellbeing. It's just that you also need to be open to the idea that simple, natural remedies may be able to solve some of your complex problems.

And remember that stories and anecdotes are super-important too, unless they're crazy. Hey... I was listening to a story this week about therapy for Depression and addiction, through the use of strong hallucinogenic drugs like LSD or magic mushrooms. There will never be a DBPCS on LSD therapy, but apparently the results are encouraging. If you don't want to go down that path, which is understandable, give my methods a try. Just because something doesn't have a DBPCS, doesn't mean it doesn't work.

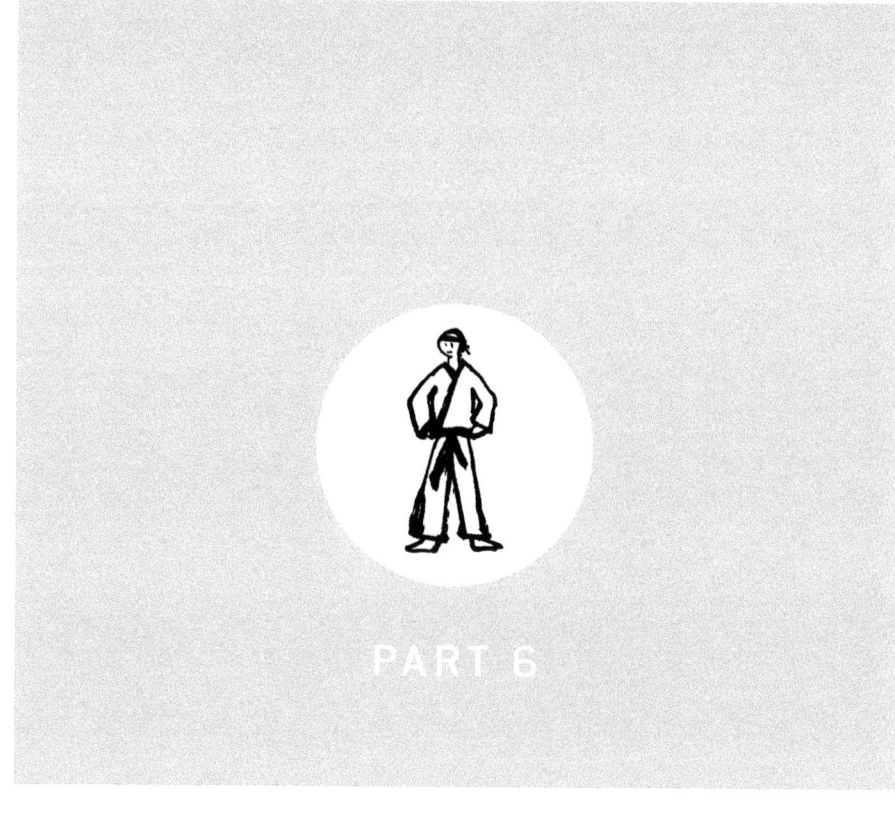

PART 6

SUMMARY + WHAT TO DO

CHAPTER 21

A Bit of Philosophy

I've really tried hard to steer away from this subject because most people think Depression is linked to philosophy (or psychology); things like, 'are you on the right path?' or 'did some external event lead to the cause of your Depression.' 'Do you have too much stress in your life?' 'Is the world against you?' As you know by now, I don't subscribe to that view. I believe Depression is almost entirely biological. Having said that, here's a bit of philosophy that may help.

Mr 90%

Let me introduce you to Mr 90%...that's me! I'm closely related to Mr 80%, Mr 70%, Mr 60% and Mr 51%. I'm totally unrelated to Mr 100% (could be a Mrs or a Miss). The thing is we're all, and in my opinion should be, related to Mr 51% to Mr 90%. When we fall outside this range, that's where things seem to go wrong. This is about the best we can aspire to. We all fall into the less than Mr 51% area from time to time, and let's call that the 'bad luck' category...not a great place to hang out. But even if you find yourself there, it rarely lasts because it's just so hard to maintain.

In anything you do, I believe you should aim somewhere between Mr 51% and Mr 90% - that will do.

I reckon people who have and maintain Depression, are often wanting to be near the 100% range. Human beings love to feel that 100% is the place where good, wealthy, and beautiful people live. WELL THEY DON'T! They live with the rest of us, just trying to cling on and survive the best they can. Get today done with, so we can move on to tomorrow. After that's over, we move on to the following day.

But there are a few of us, not too many, like surgeons and anaesthetists, who must get everything right 100% of the time, but only during their working hours. Outside of surgery, they just get on with life. Whenever I get shit wrong, which is a daily occurrence, I'll tell someone that even though I thought I got it right, it didn't turn out as I planned. I think it's called the human condition. Recognise and admit your mistakes to yourself and others, you'll be surprised how many people make them.

As one of my favourite philosophers (Jordan Peterson) says: *"Life is suffering. Your aim should be to reduce that suffering for yourself and others. That's good enough."*

When it comes to Depression, I'm speculating here, I believe many people who are the most likely to have the condition, aim for more than 90% in some aspect of their lives. Whether it be the cleanliness of their house, or the spread they prepare for guests, the standard they demand of themselves at work, the standards they believe they deserve at work, their sport, their family, their children's education - nothing is ever perfect. Once they realise and accept this revelation, it just makes life so much easier.

The thing is, when you attempt to 'perfect' any aspect of your life, you're setting yourself up for problems, and Depression is one of them. There's an awful lot of it around today, which is why we have so many rules - for example, things you can and can't say, so many signs on the highways, many workshops advising us how to live, and so many vegetarians. There's a level of 'perfection' to be achieved in these movements or philosophies. Look, you probably know by now that I'm a bit 'anti' vegetarian. There are many reasons behind this. But let's not digress. How about a vegetarian that eats meat occasionally? Is he or she suddenly excluded from the vegetarian club? Yes they are, but why? It's because the club doesn't allow digression from perfection. I became a vegetarian once when I was in my late twenties. My rule was: Vegetarian at home, but when I went out to eat, I'd choose a steak. My thinking was that a restaurant served quality meat, and cooked it far better than I would. So you could say I was 90% vegetarian … that was good enough for me. Today there's a crazy movement called 'Vegan'. Absolutely no products they consume come from an animal. So, vegans are a club striving for perfection. This is how they differentiate themselves from vegetarians, who in their view, aren't trying hard enough. Vegans won't even eat honey because the bees are animals, and that would be stealing from them. I mean seriously, where does it end? Anyway, that's not my point. The point is that as soon as you aim for 100% in any aspect of your life, you set yourself up for failure. And I hate the word 'should'… I'm not in the 'should' business. Just love and accept yourself as you are, and the world as it is - very imperfect - and loving it.

Aim to get things about right, much of the time, and you'll be happier. Don't strive to rid your Depression forever, just aim for one day without it. When that works, look for another. Then see if you can string a few of them together.

That leads me onto the next section...

Sacrifice

Let's start gently. Do you know why medicines usually taste so bad? It's not because of the stuff they're made of. Historically, people believed that if a medicine tasted like shit, it must be good. No pain, no gain, as they say. Well that tradition continues today, though children rarely fall for it. Mary Poppins was right…'Just a spoonful of sugar makes the medicine go down'. Anyhow, let me frame this in a way that hopefully makes sense to people who suffer from Depression. Why would you want to do anything that makes you feel worse, before it makes you feel better? You're feeling pretty shithouse and then some idiot tells you to give up meat, alcohol, smoking, or something else that you enjoy. I mean it's bad enough living with Depression, let alone ditching the only pleasures that make your life worth living! Then they suggest you eat Kale with every meal… please, spare me. This is a religious philosophy. It has no basis in reality.

Here's the 'do-gooders' recipe for relieving Depression: Get up at 4am, do yoga in the forest, make a kale and almond milkshake for breakfast, clean the house, and put your life in order. Then read some religious text and meditate until lunchtime. Practise mindfulness and be at peace with nature and your family. Eat well, tidy up the house and hit the pillow knowing that you've done your best. Hopefully after two or three months, you might feel more relaxed and start to come good. The prescription is all about sacrifice and moderation.

Now here's my prescription: Get up when you can. Go to the beach or just get out in the sun. Have some scrambled eggs and bacon with loads of butter and salt for breakfast. Go for a walk. Have a steak and three veggies (however you like them) for lunch with a glass or two of your favourite wine. I'd say watch a bit of afternoon TV, but it usually sucks. Indulge yourself at dinner without overdoing it, don't watch too much TV, and do something you enjoy with your evening.

Try it my way for the first day, and their way the next. Compare the difference. I'm pretty sure you'll feel better on 'my' day.

I'm not saying this is a recipe for longevity, purpose in life, or anything. Just saying I'm pretty confident that 'my prescription' is a good pathway out of Depression.

The only time you can indulge yourself is when you're alive, so don't spend your whole life in sacrifice and denial, waiting for some nirvana in Heaven. Live now!

In relation to sacrifice, you needn't experience a guilt, denial, or self-flagellation trip to cure your Depression. If you start consuming something your body likes, and usually food tastes better with plenty of salt and butter, your body should respond almost immediately.

For example, almost everyone could do with a shot of vitamin D from the sun. Go and get some good, quality sunshine for twenty minutes on a glorious day, without sunscreen, and you should feel it straight away. It won't cure your Depression, but you will feel a bit better.

And if you can consume some cod liver oil, or another good quality oil with Omega 3 and vitamin D, you should feel better too. Sacrifice is a religious concept. Just do good things that your body enjoys and it will respond quickly. You don't need to feel worse, before you get better.

'Survival' is the Only Rule

If you don't follow this one rule, none of the others matter. I read about a guy who became a hopeless heroin addict after his wife's death. He claims that heroin saved his own life. It gave him a reason to get up every day and carry on. More heroin today, meant that he could survive until tomorrow. The heroin gave him a driving force, something to live for, a reason to survive. I mean it's a very high risk method, but it worked out – for him. Today he has a good job and lives a reasonable life.

You only have one duty in life and that's to yourself, to survive. So if that means breaking every other rule that you know (without harming others) and it makes you feel better, then do it.

I've known Depression sufferers who take a summer holiday and tell me how much better they feel after it. They put this down to factors like the removal of work stress, or the difficulty of modern family life. But the real reason they feel good is because they received more sun, ate better food, often drank more alcohol, and indulged themselves. They spent more time outdoors and enjoyed good food. I've tried to explain this reality on numerous occasions, but they won't have a bar of it. 'Stress relief' they say…but they're wrong. Spending more time 'surviving' is what makes them feel so good.

Longevity

There are many things I've mentioned in this book that are contrary to what you've been told by the medical profession in regard to increasing your longevity. A great example is 'sunshine'. Almost everyone else in the world is warning you to cover up, but I'm telling you exactly the opposite…and I'll take that criticism.

Remember, I'm not here to help you live to a hundred. I'm only here to improve your life and rid you from the scourge of Depression. You may well say, 'yes, but if I stay out of the sun and drink less wine, I'll live to eighty-five instead of thirty, like the Romans used to'. Fair enough comment, but fact is, you'll only live to eighty-five due to the following; availability of calories, sewage systems, sanitation systems, clean water, heating in winter, clean health care, communication and transport, warm clothing, fewer wars, less violence, education, and the list goes on; almost none of which are provided by the medical profession. Cleanliness in hospitals for instance, was put forth and championed by Florence Nightingale, who wasn't a doctor. Washing of hands in hospital environments, was introduced by a doctor in 1850. His thesis for antiseptic policies and hand washing were rejected by most of his peers for many years after the proposal.

We accept and revere doctors' advice that will extend our lives by a few years, but we disrespect the ancient traditions of food, its preparation, and the availability of calories and nutrients. We seem to think that we can have our cake, and eat it too. In many instances we can, and if you manage to get away with it, I take my hat off to you. The thing is, by ignoring traditional practices, our gut health, and hiding away from the sun, we often sacrifice the quality of our lives. Believe me, I'd love to live to eighty or a hundred, it's a noble cause, but if I knew that would involve sitting at home, staying out of the sun, avoiding driving a car, not getting drunk, smoking cigarettes, dancing, or possibly contracting the occasional disease, I'm absolutely certain I'd choose 'excitement' over 'longevity' every time.

I subscribe to what I call 'Keith Richards' doctrine'. He didn't name it, I did. If I'd been to that many parties, loved so many women, been a member of the legendary Rolling Stones, and died at fifty, I think I'd be satisfied with that. But he's seventy-six now and still going strong. Sure, it's sort of a modern miracle, just an anecdote, but anecdotes are worth paying attention to.

With modern engineering, and a little help from medical science, your possible lifespan has increased from forty, to eighty years. If you do everything that modern medicine tells you to do, you might extend your life from seventy, to eighty years. If you ignore them and do whatever you want to do, you may only make it to sixty-five or seventy-five. It's worth consideration, but does it really matter? Follow my prescription, get rid of Depression and live your available years to the fullest. One of my favourite philosophical thoughts comes from a great businessman who on his deathbed didn't say, "Hey, I wish I'd spent more time at the office." Take your life outdoors whenever possible, eat fabulous food, indulge yourself and forget what most modern medicine tells you. Modern engineering has done far more for your longevity than medicine has.

There's a whole lot more to this and another book could be written, but let's take a more clinical, or mathematical view on longevity.

Primarily, our lifespans have improved because of successful birth rates. Not just for babies, but for women as well. The second reason is due to advancements in child health up to the age of twelve years, when to some extent they can fend for themselves.

The things I recommend may not increase your longevity by much, I'll give you that. Then again, recommendations from medical professionals regarding staying out of the sun, eating less salt and meat, keeping cholesterol low etc, won't increase your lifespan by very much either. And these recommendations are quite un-natural and for the most part, unproven.

As far as conspiracy theories go, there's certainly a big one out there… the pharmaceutical profession want to keep us just sick enough to be reliant on their products, and they 'use' the medical profession to help them. Can't say that I subscribe to this theory, but it isn't unreasonable.

Mindfulness

I have some respect for the mindfulness movement but I think that when you're suffering from Depression, it's really hard to get into these meditative, mind-changing disciplines. I know that I resisted it at the time.

What I don't have much respect for, is the way that mindfulness is taught (to be fair I haven't experienced all of it). But I've figured out a version of 'Mindfulness for Dummies'.

So mindfulness is, and should involve paying attention to the 'real thing' right in front of you. In other words, being 'present' in the moment. I'll give you an example. We see many people crossing the road these days, with their heads stuck in their mobile phones...you may be one of them. If a herd of charging buffaloes were coming at them, I wonder if they'd think, "Gee…I should google the weather forecast for today." NO! Pay attention to anything that has the potential to kill you. It's the same with anything you do. That 'real thing' which represents a threat, or an opportunity, that's right in front of your nose, deserves your full focus.

The mindfulness I've witnessed concentrates on touch, temperature, muscles, and breathing, as techniques for being present in the moment. Thing is, all of these processes are automatically taken care of by your body. You don't need to pay that much attention to them, unless something threatens your safety. You only have to focus on temperature when it represents a threat, like it's too cold or too hot, but the rest of the time it doesn't deserve that much thought. Your body will regulate your internal temperature for you, and there's not much you can do about that.

If there's a person in front of you with an axe in their hands, they deserve your attention, even if it's only your neighbour coming to chop some annoying branches. That's mindfulness. Pay attention to things that are important, especially things that are right in front of you. Pay attention to your own survival.

The Two Experiments

This is so easy...it's like taking candy from a baby, so to speak.

Let's say you, or someone you know has Depression. If either of you live in Australia, you're usually entitled to four weeks holiday per year.

Take two weeks off and test my two experiments.

I prefer Experiment (1) first, then the second, but it doesn't matter much. It's just two weeks out of your life, which, if you suffer from Depression is nothing, right? Besides, time has little meaning for those with Depression - I know, I've been there. You can do most of this at home and it doesn't require a journal or having to be disciplined, though you can if you want to.

Experiment (1)

- Breakfast every morning for the week: bacon and eggs, or something similar.

- Try for 1.5 hours of morning sun with no sunscreen or eyeglasses. Don't get sunburned, but push it to the edge.

- The balance of your daily food should consist of grass-fed meat and long-cooked vegetables.

- Consume plenty of salt; at least one full teaspoon more than you'd generally put on top of your food. A suggestion: Mix it in with a litre of water and drink that during the day.

- Drink water; aim for around two litres per day. Rainwater if you can, or Perrier as a second choice. Third option is to use tap water, but filter it and add some lemon juice, not heaps, just a few drops per glass.

- Don't eat any fast food during this week. If you're craving a burger, make it yourself. Get a sourdough roll, use grass-fed mince meat, grass-fed butter, and the best quality salad you can find. If you want pizza, make that yourself too. Basically spend time on yourself and just look after you.

- Drink at least two glasses of red wine per day.

- Take a walk for between fifteen and thirty minutes a day.

- Dig in the garden for a while, get dirty.

- Take some probiotics every day. Buy the good ones from the refrigerator.

- Take a spoonful (or two) of prebiotic fibre every day; Slippery elm powder, or apple pectin. You should be able to get it cheaply at the supermarket.

- Have some cod liver oil every day; liquid or capsules, it's up to you.

- Aim for eight hours sleep a night. Keep screen time to a minimum (say three hours a day, or less).

- Limit your exposure to harsh chemicals like soaps, detergents, and fluoride. Keep your shower water temperatures down to about 40 degrees.

Now, after the week, consider how you feel. Obviously there's no measurement protocol. I suggest calmly taking notes (mental or otherwise) from time to time during the week, to see if/when you feel more, or less depressed.

Experiment (2)

For this week:

- Have cereal and toast for breakfast.

- Use margarine, not butter.

- Whatever you eat, try to reduce your fat and salt intake as much as possible.

- Eat plenty of salad.

- Stay out of the sun, but if you must go out, cover up with sunscreen on all exposed skin areas and apply twenty minutes before exposing yourself.

- In short, observe all conventionally recommended health guidelines. Take a multivitamin tablet if you want to.

Now see which experiment was the most successful for you. My strong bet is number one!

CHAPTER 22

Recipe for Curing Depression

Little Things Matter

There are hundreds, possibly thousands of little things that have changed in our lifetimes. Running water, air travel, medicines, vaccinations, commoditised food, electricity, refrigerators, and chemicals, just to name a few. They're things we've taken for granted and generally enhance our lives. Our bodies, though highly adaptable, take many years to fundamentally change. A great example of a big change is the availability of calories and food of almost unlimited types and amounts. Only a hundred years ago food types were limited to seasonal foods and their availability was also limited. My wife has trouble digesting coconut, especially coconut oil cooked foods. She commented on how strange this is; I disagreed, pointing out the fact that I'd be surprised if many people in Germany (she is German) had even heard of a coconut a hundred years ago, let alone eaten one. It would be equally as 'strange' if she liked it, and it agreed with her.

We've basically replaced many natural things with un-natural counterparts. The sun has been substituted with electric lights, we've replaced growing our own vegetables with packaged and processed food…and on it goes. I don't want to go back to the dark ages, neither do you, but you have to grant me Newton's Third Law - 'For every action there's an equal and opposite reaction'.

Just one of the downsides to this modernity is Depression. There are others of course like diabetes, obesity, anxiety, perhaps cancer…it's a very long list.

Now one thing I'll inevitably hear is, "How did some dumbo engineer from Queensland in Australia, discover the link between Depression and gut health, when all the smart people in the world couldn't figure it out?" The answer is too complex I'm afraid, and that would require another book. The short answer is that I'm not the first to figure it out. But maybe I'm the first person to…(1) Work it out; (2) Actually cure myself by this method; (3) Admit to myself that it's what cured my Depression; (4) Have the time and money to research it; (5) Take the initiative to publish it; (6) Not fear my findings, my peers, or rely on an income stream that requires a drug or some study to validate it.

All I can absolutely honestly say is that this worked for me, and I wanted to know why. Then naturally, I wanted to tell everyone about it. I genuinely recognise that I'm not special, and I know others can benefit from my journey. Winston Churchill apparently said, *"Men occasionally stumble upon the truth, but most of them pick themselves up and hurry off as if nothing ever happened."*

So here's a summary of what we've covered…but more importantly, what YOU can do with this information.

Depression is caused by a lack of neurotransmitters. Serotonin is the main action in this space. It's made in your gut (mostly) by bacteria that live in your gut.

Many of us disregard our gut and abuse it by feeding it poorly, and/or killing bacteria with antibiotics and antimicrobial chemicals.

We can often help alleviate Depression by taking antidepressant drugs, but they don't solve the fundamental problem. And that problem is making more serotonin through food consumption and gut bacteria.

My Fundamental Recipe for Fixing Depression

You can make more serotonin by feeding yourself probiotics and prebiotics. I prefer not to say which products are best. Instead, I suggest you see a naturopath and ask them. They're professionals in this space. My only caveat here is that if you have to purchase hundreds of dollars worth of products or tests, be certain that they're beneficial to your health, not just someone else's pocket. Having said that, if you suffer with Depression, it makes good sense to have a comprehensive analysis of your poo sample. It will reveal which gut bacteria you are lacking and which prebiotics to feed them. The test could even indicate which parasites/bad bacteria you need to get rid of. But don't take too many supplements at once, otherwise you wont know what does what.

If you can't afford expensive products, just try some probiotics and prebiotics from your local pharmacy. After all, they're legally sanctioned products, so it's very unlikely that they'll do you harm.

Consume high-value unprocessed food like grass-fed meats, organic vegetables and tree-ripened fruits. Limit fast food to a minimum and do as much home preparation as you can.

Be thoughtful about how much sunshine you receive. In the northern hemisphere, for much of the year, it's impossible to overdo sunshine. In the southern hemisphere, ensure you're getting some unadulterated sunshine frequently. Forget about skin cancer...live for today, not tomorrow.

Also consider your water supply. Have mineral water when you can. Be aware that pH is important.

Be kind to yourself. Overindulge occasionally. Life isn't meant for constant sacrifice. Be thoughtful about yourself and your family. Don't just comply with vaccination schedules and medical alerts, do your own homework and find out the risks and benefits.

Get plenty of salt.

Use the internet for your health's benefit, not just to buy a nice pair of shoes or cheap underwear. Don't swallow everything you're told at face value. Make sure you drill down and find the real answers, the gritty, ugly stuff that no one wants to hear. Are vaccinations good for you? Are they all good? Is vegetarianism beneficial for your mental health? I don't know your answer. What I do know is that it takes hours and hours of research to find the answers that you seek, and it's unlikely to be the solution that you originally set out to find. Run some simple experiments. Being honest with yourself is one of the hardest things that you'll ever encounter. In this book I've endeavoured to help you with that. I challenge many 'normal protocols' because they must be questioned.

We'll take cholesterol as a subject to help demonstrate my point above, in regards to research and being honest with yourself. For many years I've struggled with the cholesterol question. Australia has one of the best health systems in the world. We spend over 20% of our subsidised medicine budget on cholesterol-lowering drugs. Apparently this cholesterol business is so dangerous, we spend oodles of money on drugs to lower it, and attempt to reduce it in our diets. On a vegetarian or vegan diet (cholesterol free) you can still have high(ish) cholesterol levels, because your body makes this substance. It's strange to think that after millions of years of evolution, our bodies still have this little poison-making factory within us. Maybe cholesterol is really important. Maybe we're not being told the truth about this substance. You'll certainly come across many articles relating the use of statin drugs (cholesterol-lowering drugs) to Depression. If your cholesterol is high, you'll generally be prescribed a statin drug regardless of any underlying mental health issues. There are an awful lot of physical medicines prescribed that 'attempt' to lengthen your lifespan, regardless of your 'quality' of life. So the aim of most modern medicine is to allow you to live the longest life possible. But is that really your aim? Shouldn't your aim be to live the most interesting and satisfying life possible, free of constraints about how you live that life? I don't have your answer. Obviously there's a balance here, but I can't answer that for you. In this context I'm suggesting that if Depression is reducing your quality of life, concentrate solely on that. Forget that you're overweight, have high cholesterol, maybe drink too much, or worry that you may die sooner than your neighbour. Be very cautious about what you put in and on your body, including prescription medicines and concentrated supplements. Concentrate solely on your quality of life. Once you're free from Depression, then work on living to a hundred.

For the elderly these days, once regular medicine gets hold of them they're taking between five and twenty different tablets. This is to help keep them alive, regardless of how long they've already lived. Many of them reside in retirement homes where younger people (like in their 60s) come to entertain them with song and dance shows. Sadly, they have limited time to enjoy these visits because they have to get back to their poor quality diets and administered medicines. Rates of Depression in aged care are staggering; around 50%.

Their diets are substandard and I'll bet their gut bacteria are too. Even though each medicine they take has been approved for its particular use, no one has conducted placebo-controlled studies on people taking all these drugs in combination. The elderly are little more than uncontrolled experiments and money machines for pharmaceutical companies. I'm not saying that I have the answer here, but providing them with a quality diet would do way more for their health and reduce the soaring cost (to someone) of the medicines they ingest.

Spend your money on quality food rather than substandard food and expensive medicines.

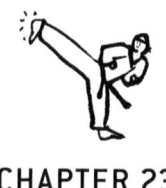

CHAPTER 23

The Studies and Articles

These are just some of the significant studies and articles that I've researched for this book:

- *The Framingham Study*
  A diet and lifestyle study of thousands of people; it has been running for sixty years. Framingham debunks many of the accepted truths surrounding diet and lifestyle.

- *Univ Tel Aviv - How antibiotics influence the chances of getting Depression.* The patients studied were 200,000 English people. You don't have to be in England to gather the data and analyse it.

- *PIP (Probiotics in Pregnancy).* A series of studies in New Zealand where probiotics were given during and after pregnancy and positively influenced the health of babies and their mothers. It revealed a lower incidence of Post-natal Depression, anxiety, and colic in babies.

- *Professor John Cryan* (Ireland) who studies probiotics and their influence on human and animal behaviour.

- An English study comparing cancer rates, in particular bowel cancer in vegetarians and non-vegetarians.

- *Effect of Probiotics on Depression: A Systematic Review and Meta-Analysis of Randomized Controlled Trials.*

- *Dr Stephanie Seneff* is fascinating; more of a data analyst and certainly an expert in Vitamin D research. She has also performed Meta analysis on Gout research. It's not very interesting to a Depression sufferer, unless you have Gout of course.

- There's a great lady named *Cate Shanahan* who was a nutritionist for the LA Lakers basketball team. She's good.

- The *'Bulletproof Coffee'* guy; he's clever but misses a lot of stuff too.

- *Jordan Peterson;* seriously knowledgeable but also lacks the biological stuff in relation to Depression.

- *Cristine Cronau;* she wrote *'The Fat Revolution'.*

- *David Gillespie* who wrote *'Sweet Poison'* amongst other titles.

- *Escherichia coli:* Enhances bioavailability of serotonin in gut tissues through modulation of synthesis and clearance.

- Interest is growing to use bifidobacterial strains (such as Bifidobacterium infantis 35624) as psychobiotics, which are *"live organisms that, when ingested in adequate amounts, produce a health benefit in patients suffering from psychiatric illness."*

- ITF is an example of well known prebiotics. Inulin naturally occurs in fruits and plants such as chicory roots, wheat, onion, banana, garlic, and leek, but is generally extracted from chicory roots on an industrial scale.

- *The International Scientific Association for Probiotics and Prebiotics* is a non-profit organization dedicated to promoting the science behind probiotics and prebiotics. ISAPP participates in science-based written and oral communications and responds to emerging scientific issues regarding probiotics and prebiotics.

- *Psychobiotics: A novel class of Psychotropic: Biological Psychiatry*. Nov, 2013. (Epub document).

- *Stress & Anxiety Dampening Effects of a Probiotic Supplement Compared to Placebo in Healthy Subjects 2018*. Front Immunology. 2017.

- *Fructose: A Dietary Sugar in Crosstalk with Microbiota Contributing to the Development and Progression of Non-Alcoholic Liver Disease*. PubMed.

I've read a lot of books that influenced my research as well:

- *The Plant Paradox*, by Gundry.

- *Dr Ted Obryen*.

- *Dr Oz* - some stuff about iron.

- *Richard Wrangham* who wrote a book about evolution, fire, and protein

- *The Power of One* - a fabulous inspiration by Bryce Courtenay.

I've been inspired by all sorts of people and publicly available resources. I have also done my best to acknowledge them, but how do you do everyone justice? You just have to search for yourself... look at studies, do your own experimentation, and hope it works for you.

My hope is that I've given you the tools to work it out. You probably won't just GET OVER IT, but I certainly hope you do.

Your body is trying to tell you something and you must give it your attention. This call for help is <u>not</u> in your head, it's in your GUT!

APPENDICES

APPENDIX 1

This may well be the first ever appendix about 'the appendix'. An appendix is described as something additional or extra.

Please read on...

The appendix is an organ that's often removed when it becomes inflamed (just like tonsils) and it doesn't seem to have any effect on us. Unlike removing a kidney, liver, heart, lung, or any other 'essential' organ, the appendix seems to be something that we don't badly need. We appear to function perfectly well without it. Translating from Latin, it means something 'added', or 'hangs off the side', but isn't necessary. From my reading and research for this book, I found contrary information, and I agree with the theory suggested below.

Normally, the appendix is situated in the lower right abdomen. Its function is unknown. One theory is that the appendix acts as a storehouse for good bacteria, 'rebooting' the digestive system after diarrheal illnesses. Other experts believe the appendix is a useless remnant from our evolutionary past.

The Appendix is a Storehouse for Bacteria

Just like us, when our ancestors were sick from time to time, particularly from food poisoning, they had to purge the gut in order to rid the invading poison or organism. This could be achieved by pooing it out, vomiting, or both. A great number of good/beneficial bacteria were also expelled, which then needed to be replenished from the appendix. If they survived, and hopefully they did, those bacteria had to be replaced quickly, especially when calories were so scarce.

In the modern world we take an antibiotic for these bacterial invasions. Antibiotics have only been widely available for around fifty years. It's quite possible that antibiotics not only kill bacteria in our gut, but also kill the bacteria stored in our appendix.

I've not seen any meaningful statistics about the prevalence of Depression in people after the removal of their appendix, so don't be alarmed if you no longer have one. Its removal can be a life-saving operation at times.

If you suffer from Depression though, have taken numerous antibiotics, and had your appendix removed, then my suggestion is to pay attention to your gut health. Do your best to get some good bacteria into your colon.

Why do people Kiss?

Because it's much more fun than licking one another's butt! Only dogs do that…and I'm guessing they aren't great kissers anyway. They don't have full, rosy lips like Kim Kardashian either, so there's a second reason.

The theory behind it is this: Dogs lick one another's butts because they're transferring good bacteria. Humans also swap bacteria when they kiss. In both cases it's instinctive. I much prefer the human method, but I try not to judge.

Antibiotics and Weight Gain

Why do farmers sometimes add antibiotics to animal feed?

The 'official reason' is that when many animals are together in close proximity, antibiotics are good for the health of the animals. The antibiotics stop the spread of disease throughout the area. And that may be the case. Besides this, the 'real reason' they add antibiotics to the animal feed is because farmers know the animals gain weight faster with antibiotics. The quicker an animal puts on weight, the sooner it can be taken to market and the more efficient the feed use becomes. In other words, more profit to the farmer. I do admire farmers, it's a tough game, but the reality is that they have to be good at making money. They may not always dress to impress, but they're far more switched-on than they look.

There are plenty of studies that show, if you take bacteria from healthy, skinny animals or humans, and put those bacteria into heftier animals (or humans), the latter become slimmer.

Yep, there are bacteria that can make you slimmer. The weird thing is … it doesn't seem to work in reverse. As usual, I have a theory on that. I'd suggest that overweight people don't have bacteria to add; they're lacking in bacteria. Whether that's a particular type, or just the diversity of it, we don't really know because the science is too new. But we'll get there. The point in relation to this book is that bacteria are really important. They do many amazing things and you'd be wise not to ignore them.

Akkermansia muciniphila

This is a long name for a bacterium found in your gut. Akkermansia derived from the name of its discoverer, Akkermanis (not to be confused with the long-haired Australian football player). Muciniphila relates to mucus, you know, snot … not snot in your nose, but in your gut. The gut is lined with a layer of mucus that needs to be cleaned, removed, and replaced constantly.

Akkermansia muciniphila is a bacterium that feeds off this mucus. The mucus then gets 'turned over' and fresh mucus is laid down. Why do you care to know this? People who are slim appear to have a lot more Akkermansia muciniphila than larger people. It's quite possible, and I'm only speculating, that antibiotics knock out a lot of this bacteria. So why don't we just make a probiotic pill with Akkermansia and solve the obesity problem? Because we don't know how to yet - the science is relatively new. We also don't know if the pill would survive in our system, get to where it needs to go, and start doing its job. These things take years to develop, even when we know the basics and someone is willing to take on the research. Then of course you have the problem that your discovery may not be able to be protected by patent. So all of your research could be lost to another corporation or the general public.

Getting back to the story... I know this doesn't have a lot to do with Depression. The reason I'm mentioning it is because bacteria do many things that are useful to us. We're just scratching the surface of understanding this hidden world of bacteria. What is important in the context of this book is that bacteria are awfully important, and you should try to take care of them. I've probably said this fifty times over by now, but I can't stress the fact highly enough. Give yourself the very best chance of fighting Depression by taking care of your gut, and your bacteria.

P.S. There are certain prebiotics (e.g. apple pectin) that target Akkermansia. If you are trying to lose weight as well as improve gut health, those prebiotics could be worth a try.

APPENDIX 2

Resilience - Emotional intelligence - Intestinal Fortitude

I'm sure you've heard about instilling resilience in children. How do we make them tougher and help them withstand the difficulties of life? Naturally, this applies to adults as well, but it's easier to teach children. There's even a measure that's often quoted today; EQ or 'Emotional Quotient'. IQ measures intelligence, therefore EQ is the emotional equivalent. It's a measure of toughness or the resilience of a person.

Here's a quote from Wikipedia:

> *"Emotional intelligence (EI), emotional leadership (EL), emotional quotient (EQ) and emotional intelligence quotient (EIQ), is the capability of individuals to recognize their own emotions and those of others, discern between different feelings and label them appropriately, use emotional information to guide thinking and behaviour, and manage and/or adjust emotions to adapt to environments or achieve one's goal(s)."*

Now I'm no expert in this field and I'm not advocating being tested, taking classes, or anything else. Toughness, EQ, or whatever you want to call it, is our ability to cope with situations and the world around us. I'd simply suggest that it's important in terms of mental health.

I've no doubt that you can learn this toughness or that it can be taught, as well as self-taught. It's a hard journey though. I'm proposing that toughness is also partly due to your diet, and more importantly your gut bacteria. Let me draw a bit of a bow here and say that EQ used to be called Intestinal Fortitude, or put in simpler terms, 'are you gutsy enough?' Do you have the guts to take on the world? There's much to be learned from these old sayings. So the clues here are 'intestine' and 'guts'. My firm belief is that gut health is a large part of your ability to cope. When you're producing the right chemicals (neurotransmitters), it allows you to better cope with your surroundings. I've personally seen this in myself, and others. I've banged on quite a bit about serotonin, but apart from the other ten neurotransmitters, the one that's applicable here is GABA (Gamma Amino Butyric Acid.) GABA is your calming neurotransmitter. When you have plenty of GABA you can calm yourself, relax, and possess the ability to make better decisions. You don't 'jump the gun' as much. You consider your options before acting. Even in a conversation, you're able to slow down and 'measure' yourself when you're less anxious. Now for argument's sake, let's say that you accept my theory about GABA. The trick is then to make more GABA. So what is it made from? Well, Gamma Amino is just a configuration of an Amino acid. That means an arrangement of molecules. Butyric Acid is an easier one though … it's butter.

Another quote from Wikipedia:

> "Butyric acid is found in animal fat and plant oils, bovine milk, breast milk, butter, parmesan cheese, and as a product of anaerobic fermentation."

So you can consume butyric acid to get your GABA, or you can make it in your gut - your bacteria will do it for you. You can also buy a GABA supplement, though I've been told they don't work too well because they don't cross the BBB (Blood brain Barrier). GABA supplements are manufactured using bacteria by the way; think I mentioned this earlier in the book. My personal belief is that the action is the Bifidobacteria; the ones that we all have, and that which children acquire soon after birth. A mother's milk is designed to feed the Bifidobacteria. So she feeds the bifidobacteria and the baby drinks it. The bacteria get fed then the baby calmly goes off to sleep (in a perfect world).

Get yourself more bifidobacteria (they're not poison after all) and you'll be calmer, less anxious, and have more EQ. Hey, give it a try, you won't suffer from the experience.

APPENDIX 3

Special Interest Groups

1. AFL Football Players and Queensland Construction Workers

For any non-Australian readers, AFL is the biggest football game in our country. The players are very highly paid and Queensland construction workers don't do too badly either. These two groups have been in the news quite a bit lately for their seemingly high levels of mental health problems. In both groups, the general consensus is that stress is a major contributor to Depression, as is working in a highly competitive 'all male' environment.

I'd like to offer some alternative contributing factors.

AFL Players: I would be looking very carefully at their diet and supplements. The fundamentals have been discussed at length in this book, but there's one supplement that I haven't mentioned yet. It's Whey Protein, or any other concentrated form of protein. In the case of athletes, these proteins are commonly used to increase muscle and bulk. Let's just stick with Whey because it's the most common. You may recall the chapter on concentration and commoditisation, which explains much of the problem here. When you concentrate something, the tendency is to alter the product for the worse. In regard to Whey, firstly; it's rarely from grass-fed animals, (strike one). Secondly; it's heated beyond the temperatures that would normally be experienced by the protein (above 40 degrees Celsius), so strike two. Thirdly: Whey powders are usually combined with many other artificial chemicals and synthetic vitamins. There's strike three. But there's nothing wrong with Whey itself per-se. It's found in cows milk and mother's milk. The problems start when the Whey is concentrated, heated, or degraded. If you read forums on bodybuilders discussing the use of Whey protein, you'll notice the large numbers reporting Depression and in particular, anxiety. My prescription for the AFL players would be (it's worth a try) to eat grass-fed meats and long cooked vegetables for a month, and avoid any synthetic cooking oils. No supplements of any kind except for some probiotics. Also, have a read of Cate Shanahan's book; she was the Dietary consultant for the LA Lakers.

Queensland Construction Workers: Again, I'm speculating here, but when you see patterns, you have to look for other patterns within those patterns. My speculation for construction workers is that it will be chemicals that they're applying or ingesting, and perhaps something they're missing out on, that causes their Depression. I'm pretty sure it will be vitamin D that's missing. Vitamin D is strongly associated with mental health issues. Construction workers are so covered up these days, it's crazy. To top it off, they apply heavy sunscreens. My bet is that they all have vitamin D shortages, and perhaps the sunscreen is poisoning them.

There's also a good chance they're using soaps and cleaning agents that are antimicrobial, destroying their skin and gut bacteria.

I had another little experiment in my mind, so I researched a bit. In looking for a common thread with construction workers, I had a look at those ridiculous high-viz shirts and clothing they wear. I mean they could cause psychological damage alone. I suppose after wearing these ridiculous outfits for a few weeks, you'd get over the embarrassment. Then I looked at the dyes that make those offensive colours. Sure enough, I found something. To make the fluoro yellowy-green colour, a chemical is used that was otherwise banned years ago. It's called PCB: Polychlorinated Biphenyl. PCBs caused numerous health problems, which have been conclusively proven. Now the PCBs used in these yellow dyes are apparently much safer because they're higher in molecular weight, or something to that nature. Fortunately, those high-viz shirts are all manufactured in China today. We all know that Chinese quality control is outstanding, so I doubt anything could go wrong there. You may recall a few years back that certain blue colour dyes were shown to cause cancer. Garments made with that chemical were removed from retailers. Almost all of those garments came from China. In Queensland in particular, there's an additional factor that comes into play. Because of our hot and humid weather, most men don't wear undergarments like singlets, so the high-viz shirts are worn directly against the skin. Due to higher perspiration rates, if there's any transmission of chemicals, it will occur more easily.

Could a lack of vitamin D, poisoning from sunscreens, harsh soaps, and ridiculous clothing be the cause of mental health problems? It's not such a silly notion.

2. Post Natal Depression

Look at the extensive PIP (Probiotics in Pregnancy) studies from New Zealand strongly supporting the use of probiotics during and after pregnancy. The outcomes from these studies speak for themselves.

3. PTSD (Post Traumatic Stress Disorder)

We're all vulnerable to PTSD if we've experience something horrific in our lives, but those who are most prone to this condition are highly trained soldiers. Now these men and women are far from weak, they're the most credentialed people that money can buy, but the problem is a huge one. So if you want to help this condition, you need the best arsenal you can get. That means high levels of gut bacteria, vitamin D/ sunshine, good levels of salt, and quality water. I don't know if it's a cure by any means, but it's a good start.

Take a look at this article on PTSD and do a google search on PTSD and Bacteria, or probiotics:
(https://www.sciencedaily.com/releases/2017/10/171025103140.htm)

APPENDIX 4

Vitamin and Mineral Deficiencies

Listen, this is a subject I'm no expert in - your doctor or naturopath is far more knowledgeable than me. However, during my research I've come across many common themes and causes of Depression; for example, iron deficiency or overload, iodine deficiency (or thyroid problems), vitamin B12 deficiency, folate deficiency, poorly functioning liver etc.

My advice is, as for the rest of the themes in this book ... give yourself the best biological basis to solve your Depression. It may be simpler than you think. In Australia, due to our excellent health cover and PBS system, many tests are free, or cost very little. In other countries, I'm no too sure.

Here's a list of tests that aren't routinely checked. You may request for your doctor have a look at them:

- Vitamin B12 status
- Vitamin D status
- Red blood Cell Folate studies
- Complete iron studies panel
- Thyroid hormone testing including TSH, free T3, free T4 and if you can, reverse T3 (rT3)
- Liver enzymes
- Glucose or HbA1C (HbA1c is an average of your blood sugar over three months).

Naturally, sodium and potassium levels are also of importance. You're hoping to be in the middle of the range at least, not at the lower end. Now if you research the internet, you'll find there are studies linking all of these conditions (being too low, or high) to Depression. I have some experience with vitamin D, B12 and Iron, so let's take a quick look at what I can suggest.

Vitamin B12

Whatever the reference range, you really want to be in the higher end of the range, not just above the lowest. Now B12 supplementation doesn't always work because most of the B12 supplements, including the one your doctor administers by injection, are synthetic substances that your body doesn't recognise. They work for some people but not others. If your B12 status is suboptimal, I'd look at consuming high B12 foods like beef, yeast, and mushrooms. There are natural forms of B12 supplements too. You can always try the one from the doctor, but I know in my case, synthetic B12 tends to have mood-lowering properties.

Vitamin D

One of the core recommendations of this book is to get plenty of vitamin D, primarily from the sun. When you have your levels checked, you want to be as close to the top end of the range as you can. This is virtually impossible to achieve if you don't get regular exposure to the sun without sunscreen, and expose your eyes as well. By all means take vitamin D supplements, but they are quite weak. You can also obtain vitamin D from foods. You need good quality fat to convert it into vitamin D-cholesterol in your body.

Iron

I'm sure we've all been indoctrinated with the importance of iron. It's essential for making blood. But when you're over the age of forty, too much iron can be a problem. It's a modern dilemma because many years ago we didn't live far beyond forty or fifty, so iron overload wasn't heard of. Now, there's even a gene mutation, only recently discovered, that predisposes you to iron overload. This won't be a problem for you until the age of forty, but even then it's still rare, like 1/200 of white Europeans. It's often referred to as the 'Celtic curse' because it's more common in northern Europeans. More likely though, if you're younger and particularly if you're a vegetarian, iron deficiency can be an issue. The remedy is to eat plenty of iron rich foods like red meat and cook on cast iron pans.

Iodine

Iodine isn't mentioned above, but it's strongly related to your thyroid gland, which is like the master metaboliser. If your thyroid isn't functioning properly (which is common enough) then you may well not be producing good neurotransmitters or getting the most out of your food supply. Iodine is so important that almost all advanced countries add iodine routinely to their salt supply. A hundred years ago iodine deficiency was extremely common, especially in areas where farming took place in low-iodine soils. These include large parts of the southern USA, Asia, New Zealand, and Australia (particularly Tasmania). In fact, adding Iodine to salt supplies appeared to increase the IQ of children by around 15 points, which is huge. From what I can make out, iodine deficiency is probably the world's most prevalent mineral deficiency, with possibly two billion people affected.

Do any of these issues on their own lead to Depression? I don't know. On the other hand, if you're low in vitamin D and B12, high in iron, have high blood sugar, and are low in iodine, then it's quite possible that your energy levels are low…maybe there's more going on. Again, give yourself the best biological chance of curing your Depression before you look at more complex issues to solve, like whether your thinking's correct, your genes are to blame, or your response to stress requires attention.

APPENDIX 5

Antidepressants

Just so you know…I'm not against antidepressants. Like antibiotics, they're wonderful drugs that save and improve lives. I think if you're prudent in wanting to help yourself alleviate Depression, the first thing you should do is consult a doctor or psychiatrist then get yourself onto an antidepressant as soon as possible. Most sufferers wait far too long to consult a physician. It's a natural human condition to not want to admit to having a problem, or submit to taking medicines. But the reality is, you need help. The newest medicines are generally the best, like SSRI medications. Personally, I don't think you should muck about with generic brands, but you can make that choice. I also advise that whatever brand you're on, stick with it, don't chop and change. They don't seem to cross over well, from observational data only.

What antidepressants won't do is 'fix' the problem. And that's fine if it's okay with you. I think they're often a wake-up call. You'll face a few possible scenarios in relation to this medication: You could go on them for a few years, they work, then you don't need them anymore. You might take them for the rest of your life. Or you could find that they work for a few years but suddenly cease working, so you need to change to a different medication. In any of the above scenarios, there's something in your diet, lifestyle, or biological health that needs to be solved. I don't feel that you can take antidepressants, go back to whatever you were doing, or consuming beforehand, and think that's the end of the matter. I strongly encourage you to start with antidepressants (if required) then have a good, hard look into other aspects of your general health, diet, or gut bacteria, to see where you can make improvements. I realise that time, money, and effort, are all against you … but don't think of antidepressants as a means to an end, rather a bridge to better health and a better life.

Now one drawback for most antidepressants is that they require time to work, say six weeks or so. By the time you finally ask your GP for an antidepressant, you're already pretty depressed and need something URGENTLY…I get that…been there! All is not lost, there's a little trick you can use. They're called benzodiazepines, though they can be a bit dangerous. Examples include Valium, Lorazepam, Clonazepam, and Alprazolam. I personally have experience with Valium and Clonazepam. If used wisely, they work quickly, within hours, and they can really turn around a bad situation. The downside is that they're highly addictive or habit forming, within only a month or so, therefore getting off them can be a problem.

I don't like Valium - it makes me a bit zombie-like. I didn't seem to care too much about anything and lacked motivation. The drug itself is over fifty years old, and today, there are better drugs available. I guess it beats being depressed though, and it's probably the least addictive of them all. I've heard that Lorazepam works well and I'm prepared to believe that. It's possibly the easiest to get off, but that's speculation. I've had experience with Clonazepam. It works quickly too, but again, is hard to get off after only a few months. You're far better to take something that keeps you stable, than battle on risking worse outcomes. I've heard of people taking Clonazepam for many years, never escalating, and leading perfectly normal lives. Alprazolam is highly dangerous. It should only to be used for short term, intense situations. It's also highly addictive.

The take home point is that if you need something NOW, try Clonazepam. It works quite well, but as I said, it's not a long-term solution because of its likelihood to cause dependency.

The thing about Clonazepam is that its main action is to calm you down. It works on GABA and serotonin at the same time.

Obviously you need to consult your doctor on these issues, but it's better to be informed of these things before you do, so you can 'steer' your GP to a workable solution. Their time is limited and they can't be expected to think of everything.

APPENDIX 6

Here are some things that I know cause me Depression, or low mood at least. Your list may be entirely different, but try to pay attention to what you're consuming, and how it makes you feel.

- Synthetic vitamin B12 (Cyanocobalamin)
- Whey protein
- Some Scotch whiskeys and most Irish whiskeys. The Scotch that works for me is Johnny Walker Black label. Generally the whiskeys that don't work cause abdominal discomfort too.
- Chardonnay - especially wooded chardonnays and Pinot Grigio
- Highly-oaked wines. There are traces of a poison called urishirol in oak, the highest amount is found in Poison Oak
- Vodka made from wheat, which is many of them
- Tonic water (but it takes a few glasses). It's the quinine.
- Paracetemol
- Cox-2 inhibitors (anti-inflammatory drugs)
- Some antibiotics
- Clove cigarettes
- Long periods without sunlight
- Highly alkaline water (again, it takes a while)
- Poor quality cooking oils (they cause sleepiness).

The point is...this list has taken me many years to compile. I don't know if they cause you any problems, but are you really looking?

APPENDIX 7

Here are some other similar diets and lifestyles that promote my beliefs.

Now I don't profess to know much about these protocols, but if my simplified methods aren't working for you, and you believe in the science, take a look at them. Be warned...they're considerably more complex.

- GAPS (Gut And Psychology Syndrome)

- SCD lifestyle (Specific Carbohydrate Diet)

- Low FODMAP diet (Fermentable Oligosaccharides, Disaccharides, Mono saccharides and Polyols)

- Paleo diet - eat like a caveman.

<u>Note:</u> These diets aren't primarily concerned with mental health, except for the first one - they're more aimed at general health.

Afterword

When it comes to diet, so many common-sense health recommendations are either wrong, or the opposite of what we've already been told. Many of them provide little, if any reliable data, so they're guesses at best, or wrong at worst. Two recommendations remain clear; sugar is bad for us, as is smoking… but that's about it. That being said, lung cancer rates and smoking rates aren't perfectly aligned by any means.

In the past we were advised that fat was bad for us, so we changed to low-fat diets. What happened? Obesity rates went up.

We were told that cholesterol was unhealthy, so we started cutting out red meat. We now eat 30% less meat than thirty years ago. We consume more fresh vegetables too. What has happened? Yep, obesity rates have risen. Hong Kong has the highest meat consumption in the world. These people aren't obese and statistics reveal a very long, average lifespan (if the mainlanders don't get hold of them).

We're informed that high fructose corn syrup and artificial sweeteners are better than sugar. We ditched sugar, then obesity and diabetes rates rose.

We're also told that salt is unhealthy, however people in the highest salt consuming countries live the longest, and have the lowest rates of heart disease. The lowest salt consuming countries reveal people with the shortest lifespans.

Apparently the sun is bad for us as well, so we all started to cover up. Rates of melanoma have continued to increase. Deaths from Melanoma have decreased due to improved detection, but the more we've stayed away from the sun, melanoma cases have increased.

During my research I stumbled across something very interesting. When Barack Obama was inaugurated, they held a grand dinner (nothing unusual there). But what was on the menu? Absolutely everything we're told 'not to eat'. So these people are possibly the most powerful, wealthy, and intelligent in the world, and they're eating all the things we have been warned not to. Doesn't make a whole lot of sense, does it? Tofu and spinach weren't being served, it was Bison, grass-fed meats, turkey, wild-catch fish, and top end cheeses. Plenty of saturated fat, nothing lean or salt reduced.

In recent times, the most significant aspect of our lives that we've changed is our relationship with food. We used to only eat for survival. The majority of people spent their days sourcing and preparing it. Now food has simply become fuel, while we spend most of our time figuring out how to acquire other things like big screen TVs, cars, houses, or recreation time. I'm certainly not berating you for doing so. We all want the good life. But here's the thing... I strongly suggest spending more of your precious time and money on what you put into and on your body. Expend your time and effort to surviving, it will make you happier, and hopefully improve your mental wellbeing.

Don't blame yourself for your Depression - you've been given all the wrong health messages. Get back to fundamentals and you'll have a far better chance of beating Depression.

One last thought... Depression has nothing to do with happiness. It isn't the opposite of happiness. Depression is a state of chemical imbalance in your body, not your brain. You can be the wealthiest person around, and still be depressed. It isn't your life that's fucked-up, it's your gut, your diet, or your general health. Everyone's life gets screwed up from time to time, and for some, it's often. That's the nature of life I'm afraid, rightly or wrongly. I didn't make the rules. Feed yourself in the best way that you can. Look after your gut, it's an easy and cheap process. Spend as much of your money as humanly possible on quality food and proper preparation. It will be well worth it.

I've spent my entire life (I'm 57) in a state of relative happiness. I was well educated and have a loving wife and family. I've also acquired more money than I ever expected (or deserved for that matter). I haven't figured God out yet, though I have come to peace with him/her. I've travelled, read a lot, shown love, and been loved. And just like you, I've experienced Depression of varying degrees. It doesn't matter whether you're a nice person or an arsehole; none of us deserve it. But like they say, 'shit happens'. Try a couple of my recommendations. I hope they work for you, as well as they did for me.

The 'S' Word

I've deliberately avoided use of the 'S' word throughout this book. It only appears once because it's a direct quote. Sometimes, this word is the ultimate consequence of the disease we know as Depression. Therefore, you must address it from every angle you can. Try my methods, I'm confident that they work, and they certainly did for me. But you won't always find the answer just from these methods alone. It's often more in depth than that, like really investigating the gut thoroughly and restoring it over a number of months. That's why I suggest that in the meantime you take an antidepressant if you have to.

Here's my little thought bubble about the 'S' word; I've been there (well almost), which means I understand how this can happen. There was a recent case in Australia where a high profile ex-sportsman drove his car straight into a tree. This would appear to be an obvious case of the 'S' word. I'm not giving any details because there's no reason to put ideas into anyone's head. What I want to share is that there's no coming back from this situation. If you feel like you've reached this conclusion, you have to do literally anything to prevent it from occurring. Firstly, don't do anything alone… don't be on your own under any circumstances.

The second step's a bit more challenging; whatever it takes for you to remain here with us, is completely acceptable (whether it's legal or not… you know I don't judge!).

So whether you're a drinker or not, buy yourself a good quality bottle of alcohol and drink it. Doesn't matter what time of day it is. Don't drive your vehicle and avoid anything or anywhere that's dangerous. Absolutely everything is permitted if the alternative is the 'S' word. Push away today's problems and launch them into the future…remember, you need to make sure there is a future.

Forget about shame, embarrassment, or any other emotion you can think of. Just be here for today and take it one step at a time. You will recover from this. I know you probably don't feel that way now, but you will. If you stick around for long enough, you'll actually fix the problem.

DO WHATEVER IT TAKES…dig a hole, paint a room, watch TV, take something that makes you feel slightly better…anything that extends your chances of making it to tomorrow, is the right thing to do!

All the very best – you don't deserve to have Depression and you are not guilty of it.

P.S. Thanks heaps for buying my book.

Ross Wilkinson

Lightning Source UK Ltd.
Milton Keynes UK
UKHW020705070820
367857UK00006B/1001